Cancer

Diary of a Daughter

A. J. King

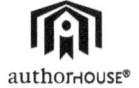

authorHOUSE®

AuthorHouse™ UK Ltd.
500 Avebury Boulevard
Central Milton Keynes, MK9 2BE
www.authorhouse.co.uk
Phone: 08001974150

First published by AuthorHouse 1/18/2010

ISBN: 978-1-4490-3709-3 (sc)

This book is printed on acid-free paper.

This book is dedicated to my wonderful dad, Brian King, who taught me so much in such a humble and unassuming way.
My love for you is eternal.

Acknowledgements

Shaun: my loving and supportive husband. Without you in my life over the last twelve years, I would not be the person I am today. I thank you for your love, loyalty, and support, even when I have had the most whacky of ideas; you deserve a medal.

Rebecca and Daniel: my two miracle babies. The doctors said we would be lucky to have children, and they were right; I consider myself the luckiest woman alive to have you both in my life. You have brought me joy from the day you were born and taught me more than any professor could have. Thank you.

Rita Pringle: the best mum in the world. You allowed me to be me and to make my own mistakes, and you were always there to pick up the pieces; never underestimate the power that you had in my life, and never listen to the criticism of others.

Ange: my little sister. How much love can a sister have for a sister? We did not always agree; you felt left behind at times, but you have played such a major role in my personal development; loving and caring for you has been a gift.

Nathan, Jack, and Emma: my nephews and niece.

You have given me the capacity to love all children. Although you may not remember, I have considered you my own over the years and, from a distance sometimes, have always had your best interests at the forefront of my mind. You are more valuable in my life than you may realise.

Louise: my best friend. We may neither talk as much as we would like nor see each other as much as we would like, but some spirits are just meant to be connected. I don't know what I would do without you in my life.

Amanda: even though you came to me for help, you have had just as big an impact on my life as I have on yours. I am inspired by your creativity enough for me to revisit mine. Thank you. And thank you for doing such wonderful illustrations for the front cover and for inside the book; you brought how I felt to life.

Auntie Hilary: I am so pleased that you are back in my life, and in such a short time you have rekindled that feeling of unconditional family love. You are and always have been special to me.

Caroline: my little cousin. I gained a sister this year when I thought I was reconnecting with a cousin. How strong is the King gene?

Alan Rowe, Roger Marsdon, Doug Brown: you were all instrumental in my life as mentors and taught me more than anyone else I can remember during my career. Thank you, because these lessons are transferable to life, and I treasure them.

Don, Jayne, Donna, Lis, Michael, Andrew, Simon, Emma, and my many other friends and colleagues at IKEA: although our time together was short, you need to know how much impact it had on my life. I was re-inspired to the point that I knew there was more for me out there, and although that brought about parting, it was the start of a new beginning for me. I learned something from each and every one of you, and I am eternally grateful.

And finally my grandads Jack and George and Nana Elsie: although you are no longer with me, the lessons you taught remain with me for the rest of my days. Always remembered with love and gratitude, thank you for your wisdom.

Introduction

This is not a story about cancer; it is a real life journey.

I started my diary to record my emotions during the most traumatic time of my life so far. Decisions were instant because time was of the essence, and at times I would rather have sat in a heap crying than writing. But I persevered as I knew that I would not be able to recapture the emotions if I had waited. So, if you haven't guessed by now, I am actually writing this introduction after completing the book. The story that you will become part of is one of love, sadness, and the reality of relationships and opinions.

The year 2009 started for me as any other year had; I was working full time as a senior manager in the retail industry with my "house husband" taking care of the mundane stuff and our children. I was happy, enjoying my job and my life. I had good relationships with family and friends, had strong self-belief and confidence, and was planning an exciting future. Then something changed; somebody challenged me and suggested that I was in denial about more than I thought. I reflected on this and decided it was work, but I was confused about what I should do.

One Sunday morning in March 2009, I was driving to work when an adult deer jumped onto the dual carriageway right in front of my car. I jerked the car left to avoid hitting the deer and crashed at 60 mph into the verge. I was knocked out and confused but did not seem to have any major injuries. An ambulance arrived and whisked me to a hospital where I was X-rayed, examined, and questioned. The injuries I sustained kept me off work for a month. I could return but would need a minimum of three months' more treatment.

Having one month off work gave me the time to really think about what it was that I was in denial about, and I set off on a voyage of discovery. I read books, signed up for online study, and started to draft a "Plan for Life."

By the time I returned to work on 1 April 2009, I had made my decision, met with my line manager, discussed my options, and left work that day on good terms. This was major. I had a limited amount of money but some big ideas; starting out on my own was scary but exhilarating and definitely liberating. I called a friend who has her own business and asked if she would give me a job for about twenty hours a week doing something fairly basic, a non-thinking job; she obliged. This would keep the wolves from the door. I signed up for a second online study course and put my Plan for Life into action. Studying, writing business plans, networking, and effective time management became my day job.

Then in June, I collapsed at work following a week

of sickness and stomach cramps. Once again, I was whisked to hospital in an ambulance for pain relief. I was diagnosed with gallstones and stayed in for a week in a morphine-induced state. Whilst in that state, I fell out of bed and put my back out, but forced myself to walk out of the hospital to get home. Another month off work followed. Nothing that had happened to me so far had stopped me from being focused or feeling positive about the future. I saw events as merely opportunities to review my plan.

On Tuesday, 7 July, I received a phone call from my stepmother, Audrey, to tell me that my dad was in hospital with a suspected stroke. I was floored; I loved my dad so much, and he had always been so fit and well, with only a few blips. I was still unwell myself and awaiting a date to go back into hospital for my gallbladder operation. I called my sister Ange to tell her about Dad, and she was distraught. My dad and her had had a rocky relationship over the last five years and had not been speaking for most of that time. I had tried to reunite them, but they were as stubborn as each other, and my dad's wife really did not like my sister. Audrey loved my dad very much but found it very difficult to share him with others who loved him; this caused resentment and grievance. Luckily, though, my sister and my dad had made amends earlier in the year at my son's birthday party and were taking small steps. They loved each other, so it was repairable.

I started to research strokes on the Internet and discovered that most people make some sort of recovery and some a really good recovery, so I felt a bit better. My mum's husband's brother had also recently had quite a severe stroke and had made a reasonable recovery. So I was at ease with the situation in that it would change my dad, but at least he would still be here.

Audrey would phone me each night with an update and some very strange stories about how he was; it sounded like he was in an alternate world, rambling about all sorts of strange events, and I became concerned. I had the strangest feeling in my gut, and there was an air of foreboding that I could not put my finger on.

Then, on 21 July 2009, the world as I knew it changed with one phone call and a diagnosis of cancer. That night I decided to document the journey, warts and all, and I already knew that I needed to make something good out of something bad. The royalties from this book will be distributed as follows:

Fifty per cent to Cancer Research UK.

Fifty per cent to my dad's five grandchildren, for their future.

The year 2009 has been the most inspiring and educational year of my life; I have learned more than ever before academically and emotionally. I genuinely believe that everything happens for a reason, and I am eternally grateful for having the time to spend with my dad, no matter how that time came about.

I am delighted to be able to share my learning with

you, and I hope that you can take inspiration from my experiences.

Life is just one big, long lesson, and we must pay attention in order to better appreciate all the people, experiences, and opportunities that will touch our lives.

We have one life; it is our duty to live it fully. Remember, dreams are your brain telling you what to wake up and do; never see events as something that should stop you but as merely a time to pause, reflect, learn, and move further forward.

Good luck on your journey.

Cancer - Diary of a Daughter

21 July 2009
9.35p.m.

Tonight I made that call.

That call to see how you were doing.

Expecting to hear "he is getting better." After all, people do improve from strokes.

I was not prepared for that.

My dad.

Not my dad.

When Audrey said, "Your dad's got terminal cancer," it was surreal.

I went into instant denial.

They must be wrong.

They can't be right.

Somebody else will come along and say it was a mistake.

I don't want to lose you.

It's 11.35 p.m., and I can't sleep.

Tears keep coming; I can't seem to stop them.

I can't stop thinking about you.

You spent a lifetime making me laugh.

I am so proud to have you as my dad.

You can't leave me.

You are too young at sixty-seven; that's not right.

I am numb, but still the tears come.

It's 11.58 p.m.; I must have been staring at the page for twenty minutes.

I know I love you, and I will treasure the time we have left.

Every day is a gift, and I will speak to you every day that you are able.

I am going to lie on the bed and stare.

The tears are still coming; they won't stop.

This world is better with you in it. What a waste!

Goodnight, Dad. I am sending the biggest hug you can imagine.

My daft, lovely dad.

12.07a.m.

22 July 2009
8.55 a.m.

Didn't sleep much last night; tears and memories kept flooding.

The sun is shining today, and I face the world with sadness.

But I will try not to cry.

I have made pancakes with the kids and had fun; they don't need to know yet.

Audrey asked me not to tell anyone yet, and I must respect her wishes.

She has made you happy, so I am grateful to her.

I remember when I was young, and you used to do big kissy time and big licky time!! You would kiss and lick my face, and it tickled so much I laughed until it hurt. I would smell of your breath, and it took ages to stop laughing. Just the threat of big licky time would start the hilarity! You were daft, funny, and I always knew how much you loved me.

I am going to study now. Must finish this diploma.

This was the year I was going to change my life and be a huge success.

I still am.

You don't need to tell me that you are proud of me.

I know.

Nothing needs to be said.

I am who I am because of you.

I watched you work hard to give us everything.

You set an immaculate example of what you can achieve in life.

You struggled with emotions and words, but I knew.

Nobody loved you more than I do.

I will write in this diary every day for you.

I will see you soon, Dad.

1.15 p.m.

Where did the tears come from again?

I have studied all morning; I have been OK, then...

I feel robbed, even though you are still here.

I will have to come and see you in the next few days.

Two hundred miles is nothing; I need some time with you.

If I feel like this, goodness knows how bad Audrey is feeling.

I need to do something!

9.18 p.m.

Walked the dogs earlier, got rid of the dark mood.

The kids have been a tonic tonight.

Could not manage any more study though. Maybe tomorrow.

23 July 2009
8.14 a.m.

Think I may have moved from denial to acceptance.

Still hurts but have stopped crying – no more poor me syndrome. This is about my wonderful dad, and I need to spend time with you.

The kids continue to inspire me today, and I await the call from Audrey to confirm diagnosis and timescales.

I am going to finish my study module today and start the next one.

With acceptance comes movement and motivation.

The year 2009 is going to be my most successful year; my dad will be proud of me.

When you worked in Saudi, Indonesia, and Oman, the most exciting part of my year was meeting you at the airport when you came home – the drive to the airport filled with anticipation and excitement, awaiting that first hug, and seeing the scruffy, long-haired, tanned man in T-shirt and jeans! Smelling of cigars and loaded with gifts – it was like going to meet a rock star. My dad!

10.18 a.m.

Reply text from Audrey; she is struggling.

I need to be strong and supportive for her; need to spend some time with her when I come down.

Completed module twenty. Starting module twenty-one and module one of my second course.

When life's problems seem overwhelming, look around and see what other people are coping with. You may consider yourself fortunate.
Ann Landers

9.37 p.m.

Spoke to Audrey. No news!

Been on tenterhooks all day and now have to wait until tomorrow.

Even harder, still can't tell Ange or Mum, which does not sit well with my values.

Spoke to Mum today and had to lie when she asked

about you.

Speaking to Ange by text – coward!

Respecting Audrey's wishes is turning out to be tough. I have nobody to talk to, and I feel bad about lying.

Don't think Audrey appreciates the position she has put me in; I will only do it until the final diagnosis is given tomorrow.

Ange has a right to know too.

Resentment and grievance should not be an issue at times like this. Why can't people see that? It's just not important.

Wonder what you would want?

I bet I never told you about being the only kid that could answer the killer question in a school quiz! The question was, "What is the capital of Indonesia?" Well, since I had been eating my dinner off a tablecloth with a map of Indonesia on it for at least a year, guess who won my team the quiz?! You taught me far more than you will ever know in more ways than you will ever know. Thanks, Dad.

Goodnight, sweet and wonderful man, I am going to tell the children tomorrow. We don't do secrets and lies in our house.

Rebecca will be devastated; she loves her grandad.

All the girls love Brian King; he is a charmer.

Because I have loved life, I shall have no sorrow to die.
Amelia Burr

24 July 2009
11.24 a.m.

I am a bit edgy today; don't know what to do with myself.

Been for a smear – easiest one ever. Seems nothing compared to what you are going through.

Leaver's assembly at 1.00 p.m. today, Becca's last day at Swarland School.

You will miss so much with my kids, Dad, but they will know what a special man you are, because I have so many stories.

I just need someone to talk to, and right now the two people I would normally phone are out of bounds; this is hard.

Then I think it's not really because what you are facing is harder, Dad.

I can't wait to talk to you.

9.45 p.m.

Finally told the kids this afternoon. Becca distraught. Dan oblivious (he is only five).

Spoken to Audrey and told her I am coming this weekend and that I am telling my mum.

She wasn't happy, but I need some emotional support!

I am angry and need to reframe my mood.

I will tell Ange when I have seen you this weekend.

25 July 2009
9.08 a.m.

Becca has begged and begged to come and see her grandad, and I have just caved. We are leaving in half an hour.

Summary of the weekend:

We arrived at 1.50 p.m., just in time for visiting, and it was great to see you. We had a laugh. Becca never shut up, and there were huge hugs all round.

Came back to see you again at 7.00 p.m. Audrey and Derek there.

You didn't look well; you were pale and tired.

Becca loved Derek.

It was a lovely night, had a chat with Audrey. All OK.

Becca and I came back to see you again on Sunday before coming home.

You told us you had cancer and shrugged it off like a sore throat. You are true to form, Dad!

Becca told you she loved you every ten minutes. So glad I brought her.

Had to leave you at 3.10 p.m. That was hard, but, like you, I am good at disguising how I really feel!!

Got home at 7.09 p.m. Dan has swine flu!

27 July 2009
9.32 a.m.

Spoke to Mum; we are going to tell Ange this afternoon.

So glad I have my mum to talk to now.

Dan had a bad night. I have had no sleep, and my back is sore. But if you can shrug off cancer, then nothing is going to bother me.

5.58 p.m.

Told Ange. Left her in tears, but she will be OK.

I talked her through it and advised her how to cope. You know how emotional she is. Well, she did you proud, and I think she will be fine.

Becca not well now; hope it's not swine flu!

28 July 2009
8.45 a.m.

It's swine flu!

Going to doc's to collect tamiflu and now coping with two sick children.

Never mind; it's keeping me occupied.

29 July 2009
10.47 a.m.

An eventful day!

Spoke to Audrey at length about staying positive for you and making things the best they can be.

Found your sister Hilary through your nephew Matthew. She sent her love. Spoke to her tonight for the first time in fifteen years.

Feel like things are getting back to normal, although there are odd little things that happen that stop me in my tracks and make me think of you.

Suppose that will always be the case. You are my dad, my hero!

Remember when you dressed up as Santa and I was able to uncover your identity? You could be covered from head to toe, and I would still know it was you. You were unmistakeable to me, Dad.

There are three stages of a man's life: He believes in Santa Claus, he doesn't believe in Santa Claus, he is Santa Claus.
Author unknown

The greatest gift I ever had
Came from God; I call him Dad!
Author unknown

2 August 2009
7.15 a.m.

I haven't written for a few days. Tried to spend some fun time with the kids, now swine flu has flown.

Studied like mad Friday night and all day yesterday, trying to make up the time that I lost when I was in hospital and the weekend I came to visit you.

Three modules left, and I will be a professional life and business coach. I will be finished in two weeks.

Then I will start the advanced diploma in NLP and counselling, then the BSc in psychology in January.

Who knew you had bred such an intelligent girl, eh?

Mum told me how proud she was of me the other day. She didn't need to, I know it. Nice to hear, though.

I have just walked the dogs. Woke up at 6.00 a.m. thinking of you and had a few tears on the walk.

OK now, though.

Received an e-mail from Hilary. So good to hear about how they are all doing! Going to reply today.

You have missed out on so much of your family over the last fifteen years, but it was your choice.

We all still love you, and if you have been happy, then there is no judgement.

Shaun and Dan are both snoring 6-foot away from me in bed. Dan sneaked in our bed at 4.20 a.m. and announced, "I'm here!" He cracks me up!!

Becca is sound asleep with Snoodle bear in her newly fitted bedroom.

She now has the most fab room – loads of storage and clothing space for my little diva.

Spoke to Moira, my business partner, yesterday. We are going to push the business launch back to October so I can visit you during the school hols.

I know I have had my own business before, but this just feels so right.

I am going to be doing something I love every day; it won't feel like work.

MPower is going to be the best training, personal development, and coaching business out there and will be international by 2011. That is my vision.

I have been writing, being creative, and it has just been flowing so easily. You don't have to have any worries about me, Dad. I now have the best boss in the world: me!

Isn't it amazing? You spend your whole life working hard and taking responsibility, and then it turns out responsibility is your ability to respond!

Goodness! I have been a bit waffly (if there is such a word) this morning!

Must have needed to say all of the things that have been on my mind over the last few days.

You know I have been fine, no tears, really strong. And then this morning I just can't stop thinking about you.

I suppose that is just how it is going to be.

I found a great quote from Paul McKenna yesterday: "If it is going to happen anyway, make it happen your way."

Do one thing for me: live!

Enjoy every minute you have; see the people you love.

Relationships are far more important than material things; they feed the soul.

I have told Audrey to ask if she needs any financial help for you to do everything that you want. So don't waste any time thinking about barriers; there are none.

Well, its 7.43 a.m., so I am going for a cuddle with my boys and a cuppa – in that order.

I won't leave it for four days again.

The most important thing you ever did for me was just be there when I needed you. No judgement; just love and support. Thank you. I couldn't ask for any more, Dad.

Any man can be a Father but it takes someone special to be a dad.
Anne Geddes

4 August 2009
9.34 a.m.

Took the kids to the pictures on Sunday to see *Ice Age 3*; laughed my socks off. Laughter is the greatest healer; it really lifted my mood.

Spent loads of time with the kids over the last two days. Dan has become my kitchen helper, and he loves cooking or making a mess, whichever way you choose to describe it.

Becca and Shaun have been taking the dogs for long walks.

Spoke to Ange yesterday; think she is in meltdown as expected, but I know she will bounce back.

My resolve seems to be getting stronger, despite the weepy morning on Sunday.

I have completed and passed four modules from two diplomas over the weekend, so I am on track with my new goal.

I may launch my business at the end of September with the planned "Confidence Building" workshops.

See a need, fill a need.
 Robots – Blue Sky Studios, 20th Century Fox

I think there is a need in the current climate to roll this out to the general public.

Haven't spoken to Audrey since Friday; we agreed to speak only when there was a change, but think I will call today to check on you.

I have managed to persuade Ange not to come this week; think she needs a bit more time, and she has no money.

Spookily, Audrey just called! The law of attraction!!

Anyway I have told her we are all coming this weekend and booked Shaun's mum for dog sitting.

Can't wait to see you again.

2.55 p.m.

Just spoke to our Caroline – so happy, my little cousin.

She may come and see you tomorrow; you are going to be made up!

Family faces are magic mirrors looking at people who belong to us, we see the past, present, and future.
Gail Lumet Buckley

A young girl looks at her dad and sees a hero. A young woman looks at her dad and sees the standard she expects from a partner. In her 40's, a woman looks at her dad with love and gratitude for being the only man to ever love her unconditionally.
Mandy King

5 August 2009
8.48 p.m.

Decided to try and liquidise all my assets and make them available for you today, so I had to do a couple of things that didn't feel great.

To hell with it. You can't take it with you!

Just had a text from Caroline saying she has spoken to you and you were chipper; I am pleased.

Been to the park with the kids today and bought them ice cream; they said it was the best day ever.

It only takes small things to make life worthwhile in the eyes of children.

Nathan may be coming with us this weekend; he wants to see his grandad.

I am going back to work next week, for a few weeks until my operation, that is; then it is another four weeks' recovery time.

What a disjointed year healthwise!

I can't stop thinking what happened with me parting company with my last employer happened for a reason.

I now have the time to spend with you, and I am so grateful.

I am tired tonight. Not been sleeping well.

Too much on my mind I think.

Going to take a time out with my friend Amanda tomorrow and have coffee and catch up.

Need to do something for me and get a couple of hours away from normality.

The picture of your face is a strong image when I close my eyes, and it is a face I love.

Goodnight.

6 August 2009
8.02 p.m.

I feel odd today.

Can't put my finger on it.

Had a lovely time with Amanda this morning. Went to Rothbury, looked at a couple of houses (from the outside), and had coffee.

Lovely.

Came home, took kids to park, beach, then tennis; I had a great time.

But I feel lost, listless, and fatigued.

Strange.

Just one of those days I suppose; I will be fine with the new day.

Coming to see you tomorrow; looking forward to it.

Going to tackle another module tonight; only four modules left to complete both diplomas.

Need to focus.

The lucky man has a daughter as his first child.
Spanish proverb

9 August 2009
10.15 p.m.

Well, we are home, having spent the weekend in Manchester.

I am weepy tonight after seeing you all weekend; you were not as well as last time.

I think I am emotionally drained.

Had lots of conversations, a few heated ones with Audrey and Derek – almost like the storming stage in teams!

There seems to be a strong will to be in control of your life, to the point where I feel you are not saying how you really feel in order to keep the peace.

I have had to have my say in a diplomatic but assertive way.

I do not want resentment and disturbance at the minute.

Why is it that people find it so hard to be objective and see others' point of view?

It always seems to be "my opinion is the law," without the ability to find empathy or understanding.

You say you don't want to play happy families to Audrey and Derek, yet I see a tear in your eye when I talk about your family.

What's that all about?

You have been hurt by people, but you have been no better yourself.

Why do we do this to each other? I wish everyone could be enlightened while those we love are still here.

Ange is your daughter, and she loves you. All the resentment is just poor communication from all sides!

Hilary is your sister, and she loves you. All the resentment is just poor communication on all sides!

Your disadvantage is that you like an easy life; you want to live with two people who seem to be incapable of seeing good in anyone and who keep the conversation firmly on the negative side. And when you don't bother to pick up the phone, why should others?

So, let me tell you how I see life and people.

Everyone is unique, special and has the ability to learn from mistakes and grow.

With the right approach, nurturing, and support, you can help others to be all they can be.

With forgiveness and gratitude replacing negativity and resentment, you feel happier.

By focusing on today and not the past, you can live your life with a smile on your face and a happy heart.

I practice this daily.

Choose your attitude and behaviour daily.

Smile when you walk down the street, and count the smiles you receive in return. Make someone's day!

When your heart and soul feel full and you focus on positives, then life feels good.

I think life is good; stuff just happens.

Deal with it, stay positive, and love.

That's all everyone has to do in order to be happy.

I am grateful for my aches and pains – they remind me that I am alive. I am grateful for Shaun getting on my nerves – it means he cares enough to bother and he isn't down the pub or with another woman. I am grateful for my kids fighting – it means they are here and safe and not being abducted by some weirdo. I am grateful for the internet – it has reconnected me with those I love and thought I had lost. I am grateful for people that complain all the time – it reminds me how easy it really is to be happy and stay positive. But most of all I am grateful that my mum and dad met because they made me, without them I would not be writing this today or have reached this point in my life. Every second counts – no matter if it is bad or good. Make it count be changing the bad stuff into good – it's easy!
Mandy King

Some people find fault like there is a reward for it.
Zig Ziglar

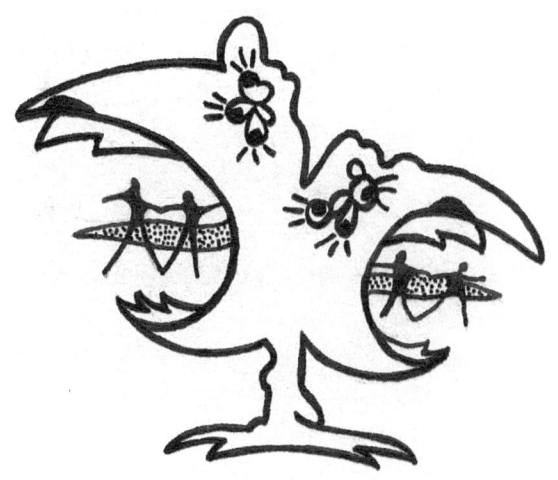

He said, she said. Illustrated by Amanda Hall Younger

10 August 2009
3.46 p.m.

I'm having a bad day!

Not grumpy, not unhappy; I just feel weird.

Sad.

Looking forward to going back to work tonight as a distraction.

Becca has gone out metal detecting with Shaun.

Dan is watching Garfield.

Remember how much I loved Garfield? You bought me the biggest Garfield known to man and loads of smaller ones. You never seemed to be there, but you always seemed to know! I thought you had special mind- reading powers, but I guess you either just took notice or asked questions. Whatever you did, those silly soft toys meant the world to me because they were from you.

Can't even find the energy or motivation to write anymore.

I feel flat like a piece of paper!

Let's hope I feel 3D again tomorrow.

10.22 p.m.

Been to work; it was a tonic.

Cried all the way home though.

This weekend has completely drained me.

I should not be forced into managing all of this bitterness at the minute.

Why oh why oh why oh why???

I am going to change the world; MPower is going to change the world.

I want you to send me a sign at my first seminar, with

an audience of over 5,000, to say you are watching, Dad.

I am in fighting mode now.

Bring it on Audrey and Derek; I am ready.

He might live in your house, but you don't know him like I do.

And neither of you will ever truly understand that connection.

You may want to watch who you talk to when you complain and attempt to devalue every member of my family; walls have ears, and I have the balls to stand up to you unlike anyone else.

Not that I want a fight at the minute, but both of you have been behaving badly for over twenty years, and it is time to stop.

You are not always right.

You are not better than anybody in my family.

In fact, your negativity and nasty comments show your true colours.

I know that nobody is perfect; but believe it or not, we learn and grow by making mistakes.

It is OK to make mistakes; in fact, it is good.

One of my regular statements is that I am never wrong; I am either right or I am learning!

You could learn something from that if you actually stopped complaining long enough.

Anyway, rant over.

This is a time for love, unity, and forgiveness.

If you can't find it in your heart to do that, I actually feel sorry for you.

I am going to bed now.

I love you, Dad.

Feelings of worth can flourish only in an atmosphere where individual differences are appreciated, mistakes are tolerated, communication is open, and rules are flexible - the kind of atmosphere that is found in a nurturing family.
Virginia Satir

11 August 2009
11.37 p.m.

Finally got my e-mails through to Caroline; it fills the gap a bit.

She is with me (mentally); the force is strong in this one!

She is coming to see you on Sunday just to remind you that there are others who love you and to talk about her mum.

I am keeping everything crossed that it is enough to soften that hard heart you have gained whilst under the influence of Audrey and Derek.

Whatever happens, you being sick has brought some much-loved people back into my life, and I am grateful for that.

I have been a bit better today. Still can't settle though.

I have a heavy heart for what you are going through and for your inability to see and acknowledge all those who love you.

Sometimes it is harder to admit we may be wrong than it is to allow love to slip away.

You are a stubborn old fart!

I wish you would drop the defence mechanisms and accept what is being offered.

Even if you don't, I still love you and always will.

The force is strong in this one too!

When the world says, "Give up," Hope whispers, Try it one more time.
Author unknown

12 August 2009
2.30 p.m.

How do I cope with the anger?

Can't sleep, restless, bad back is back, and I am really, really angry.

The educated side of me knows this is a natural process, but I feel irrational at times, and that is not normal for me.

I think the school hols are not helping. I do not get a minute to myself, and the kids are fighting all the time.

I may ask Mum to take them out for the day to give me a break.

Let's face it; it's not very often I ask.

Had to speak to Audrey again this morning; you are coming home today.

Good on her for pursuing it!

I am pleased you will be where you want to be; I hope that this will be enough for you to feel a bit better.

I am going to keep channelling the anger and grief into this diary and into my other creative work.

It is not impossible to cope under duress; it just takes focus and application.

I think I would feel better if I could get a good night's sleep. Maybe a trip to the doc's is in order if it doesn't improve – no! I will not go down that path; I am going to meditate with holosync later to see if that helps.

It's at times like this that I wish I drank, although that is not a good route either.

You are going to die, and I just can't rationalise it in my head. Well, I can sometimes and not others.

Grief is a bummer!

Think I may go and buy some comedy DVDs at Sainsbury's and watch them.

Natural healing is always the best with emotional pain; laughter and meditation – worth a try!

13 August 2009
7.54 p.m.

Well, the meditation worked a better night's sleep.

Went for a picnic with the kids at Alnmouth beach. Mum came too; we had a lovely time and a long talk.

Precious moments.

I am feeling a whole lot better today.

Spoke to Ange tonight; she feels like I did when I came back from seeing you, flat.

I am not going to write any more tonight as I am going to study and attempt to complete two modules.

Goodnight, Dad.

Sleep tight.

Wake up with the morning light.

14 August
2.26 p.m.

Not only did I complete the final two modules of my Confidence Building diploma, I also completed the final paper; stayed up until about 3.00 a.m.

That means I only have just over one module to complete the Life Coaching diploma and I am finished; I reckon by next Friday.

It is difficult to concentrate at the minute. However, once I start I find it difficult to stop until I have fully completed the module.

There have been many, many late nights.

The distraction is welcome.

I called to speak to you, but you were too ill and in bed. I have told Audrey to get you to phone me when you feel you can cope with a conversation.

There is no pressure. I would rather you speak to me when it is not a chore than force a conversation out of duty.

Audrey sounded really low today. She should not dwell on anger and negatives; every day is a gift.

My anger has subsided a little. I don't really care what Audrey and Derek think any more. In the big scale of things the only thing that matters is you.

I will not waste my time and energy on negative thoughts. As soon as I have vented I have forgotten it; wish others could do the same instead of harping on about things that happened twenty years ago.

You must live in the here and now in order to get the best out of life, and that is what I intend to do.

Wish you had lived longer so I could talk to you more; no point in wishing though, so I will focus on what I can do every day.

When I was at school I used to brag openly about you. I was the only one with a dad who worked abroad, and this made me special. I could tell my friends all the stories you told me, and they used to hang on my every word. Maybe this is where I gained my communication and presentation skills. See, I can find your influence in everything.

So much sadness exists in the world that we are all under obligation to contribute as much joy as lies within our powers.
John Sutherland Bonnell

11.05 p.m.

I have been to work and detoured via the co-op for a bottle of Asti.

Fairly harmless and like pop, but it's making me feel quite tipsy, which is good.

So many thoughts, so many people with an opinion, so many sad faces – bollocks, bollocks, bollocks!!!

Think I need a night out with friends and a damn good laugh.

I am going to waste no time on what ifs – life is too short.

I am going after my dreams with gusto and enthusiasm.

I am going to listen to no one but myself and follow my gut feeling.

So wish you were staying for the ride, but I will see you again on the other side, where we can have a ball!

Love you, Dad.

15 August 2009
9.37 p.m.

I was a bit tipsy last night. (Oops, didn't mean to reveal that. But I'm leaving it in because I want this diary to be a real reflection of how I feel.)

Had a good day today. Shaun and Mum took the kids swimming and out for lunch while I studied.

Only have my final exam to complete now; but

working for the next three days, so the goal remains next Friday.

Text from Audrey saying you had only been up for two hours today, and you were too ill to speak to me.

It's OK. You are in my thoughts every waking minute, so I don't feel deprived.

In fact, I think I have the easy job of getting on with my life whilst Audrey has to watch you fading away.

I do feel for her that has to be the hardest thing in the world to endure.

As much as I would love to be with you every day, it would break my heart to watch you deteriorate; it is devastating just seeing you for a short time when I come down.

I just want to wrap you up and cuddle you to make it better, like you did for me so many times.

I have made a list of goals for the next few weeks and really focused my mind.

Now I am almost complete with my initial two qualifications, I have to shift gear to get the business up and running.

I wish I could tell you all about it in detail. I was looking forward to doing that on your next visit.

Who knew that your next visit was never going to happen? Not fair.

I am sure that you know and you see.

I know that you are proud.

I am going to finish my book now. It's *Rich Dad, Poor Dad* by Robert T. Kiyosaki. Ten out of ten. The book has changed the way I think about money!

Love is patient, love is kind.
It does not envy, it does not boast, it is not proud.
It is not rude, it is not self-seeking.
It is not easily angered; it keeps no record of wrongs.
Love does not delight in evil, but rejoices with the truth.
It always protects, always trusts, always hopes, always perseveres.
Love never fails.
I Corinthians 13:4-8

17 August 2009
11.34 p.m.

I couldn't write anything last night. I was a bit emotional, and tears came every time I tried.

I have been fine today, and then I am a bit weepy again tonight.

I haven't heard from Audrey, so I will call tomorrow to see how you got on at hospital today.

I have been at work; that is why I am writing so late tonight.

I think I may have come up with a solution for Ange at the pub!

She has been struggling to cope with things, and guess who ends up having to support? That's right, me!

Being a mother (and father) to my sister has been hard, but it has taught me an awful lot about tolerance, forgiveness, and love.

It is such a shame that you did not have the opportunity to learn the same lesson; it is enlightening.

You know, I could be angry at you for giving up on Ange if I didn't love you so much.

You blame your parents for so much, until you have kids yourself and then you get it.

You see everything you thought was a mistake and have a newfound ability to understand why; in fact, you question if you would have even been that tolerant!

I suppose that is what it is all about, this life thing we are given: just one long learning and one light bulb moment after another.

I will miss you.

Not that I see you that often, but I know you are there.

Grief is weird; the range of emotion is just massive.

I am not used to being this out of control of my emotions.

And another thing: I have had to buy Olay regenerist eye derma-pod thingy's, because my eyes look like piss holes in the snow!

I called out for you tonight driving home in the car. I wouldn't admit that normally, but I made a commitment that this diary should be real, so there you go: I am a looney!

I am going to attempt sleep now.

Night, night.

Sleep tight.

Wake up with the morning light.

I will never forget the day you came home from Indonesia and sat me down in the living room and asked me if Mum was having an affair. My blood ran cold. Do I lie to someone I love or betray someone I love? I said no. I lied for my mum. I didn't sleep for about six weeks, and I just wanted to hug you and tell you the truth every time I saw you. But I couldn't. I'm sorry. You deserved better. I deserved better. I was fourteen years old then. I have lived with the guilt ever since, thirty years. I don't blame myself now, or anyone else. I just wanted you to know.

The guilty one is not he who commits the sin, but the one who causes the darkness.
Victor Hugo

18 August 2009
10.14 p.m.

Just arrived back from work, and for the first time in a week I did not cry all the way home and end up looking like a panda – progress!

I have had an interesting day.

Went and had coffee with Amanda this morning for three hours; she is just along the road at North Acton for a couple of weeks.

I love talking to Amanda. She and I are on the same wavelength, and she has far more about her than even she knows yet!

I am determined that she will be all she can be, with a little help from me and all of her latent talent unleashed.

I love people.

I wish you knew me better, Dad. I know you would really like me as a person and not just love me as a daughter.

There has just never been enough time.

I am determined to really know my kids; I think it will make a difference.

I feel like our family has been too judgemental and not grateful and accepting often enough.

I am pointing no fingers, as I have been that soldier!

The difference is that I am prepared to admit, acknowledge, and change my behaviour.

We waste too much time on trivial stuff, are not honest enough with each other, and gossip! I am not even going to start on how much I hate gossip.

Anyway, I am choosing my path with my remaining family, and I am going to take the responsibility to keep contact.

That is not "playing happy families" in the words of the oracle that is Derek. It is showing a genuine interest in getting to know the people who are connected to you.

Does not mean you have to like them all the same, love them all the same, or even tolerate them, but I think they all deserve the effort.

Anyway, I digress.

I have spoken to Audrey; not much to report other than you are not well.

I have also spoken to Caroline and arranged to meet her next week when I come down to see you again.

I am really looking forward to meeting up with her and bringing her to see you.

I reckon by lunchtime tomorrow, I will just about finish my final exam for my second diploma.

Wow, can't believe I have completed the two in a third of the time. It was tough, but I have learned loads.

You should have done more. You are superintelligent, but you were never encouraged.

Anyway, I am going to sign off now. I have shared my philosophies for the day. Who do I think I am, eh?

One's philosophy is not best expressed in words; it is expressed in the choices one makes... and the choices we make are ultimately our responsibility.
Eleanor Roosevelt

19 August 2009
2.34 p.m.

I have just spoken with Audrey; you have had your biopsy and are comfortable in hospital.

Apparently a cancer care nurse turned up to see you out of the blue yesterday and offered support to Audrey as well as care for you.

I encouraged Audrey to take all of the support she can get, emotional or physical.

The nurse told Audrey more than anyone has so far in terms of what will happen.

The consultants from Wigan and Christies will meet with the palliative care team to discuss how to best support you.

There may be an opportunity to have chemo. However, it will only be to stop the spread of cancer into other organs as there is no cure for what you have.

Audrey has said that she wants to keep you at home until you are really bad and then move you to a hospice.

Not once have I been asked what my opinion is; decisions have just been made.

I am sitting here with tears rolling down my face, a knot in my stomach like I have never known, and an ache in my heart so strong that you can almost hear it.

I know that Audrey is your next of kin and needs to be in control. However, it is so hard for those who love you just as much but are merely part of the communication chain.

For all sons and daughters out there who have had to go through this or will go through this sometime in your life: I know your pain.

It is a pain so intense and raw.

You sit with memories from when you were small children to being adults of these leaders in your life.

They shape you, teach you, love you even when you are bad, then let you go into the world to live your own life and make your own mistakes.

They pick you up when you fall, make it better when it hurts, and always have a hug when you need them.

They smile when others frown, brag about you to the people they meet, and exaggerate your achievements.

Then they get ill, and it is so hard for you to do the same for them.

I know some children have the opportunity to do that, and it must be hard.

But, believe me, it is just as hard being four hours away and imagining what is happening every day.

Not really being part of it; just waiting for phone calls.

Visiting every two weeks and hoping you last in between.

Praying that when the end comes, you can hold on until I get there.

Snatching moments, treasuring them, and locking them away in memory forever.

My lovely dad.

I am going to miss you so much.

I am sobbing now. I can't phone Ange and give her an update because I don't want her to feel like this.

I need to be her rock at the minute.

I will be OK in five minutes.

So, when you feel like crap, God sends kids to slide down the stairs on the dog blanket!! That brought me to my senses. Thank goodness for Becca and Dan.

You are worried about seeing him spend his early years in doing nothing. What! Is it nothing to be happy? Nothing to skip, play, and run around all day long? Never in his life will he be so busy again.
Jean-Jacques Rousseau, *Emile*, 1762

When the pain of losing a loved one hurts, let it remind you to love the living even more intensely.
Mandy King

I just had a thought.

If you and Mum were still together, then maybe this would all be easier; it would not feel so distant or remote.

It is divorce and re-marriage that puts the wedge in place.

Vying for affections, needing to be in control, resentment yada, yada.

How can someone who has been married to you for thirteen years and has no children of her own ever understand my pain?

My mum understands my pain, but she has her own husband and her own life.

I understand Audrey's pain because I have a husband I love, but she can never truly understand mine because she does not have that parent-child bond which gives you so much more understanding in life.

Then maybe I need to be more understanding of her inability and be the better person.

I will for you, Dad.

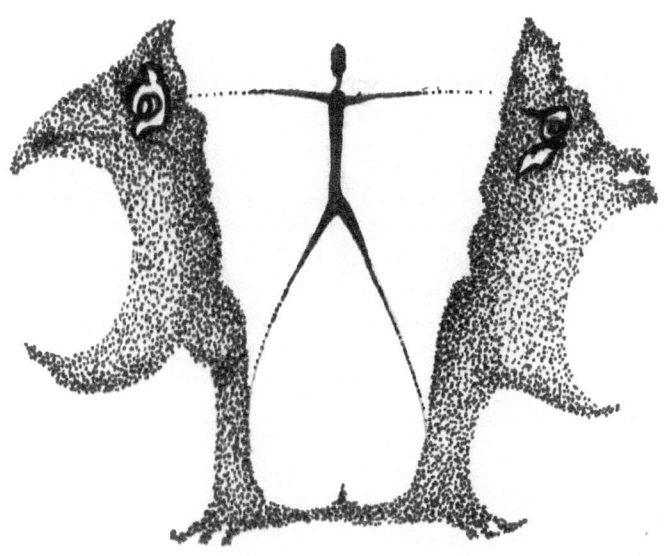

Divorce.   Illustration by Amanda Hall Younger

20 August 2009
4.23 p.m.

We have all been to Newcastle shopping for school shoes and clothes. So I would like to say AAARRRRRGGGGGGGGHHHHHHH on behalf of all parents and pray I survive mentally and financially until the small, expensive ones go back to school.

What a distraction though, I have not hurt as much today and feel OK at the moment.

It does not mean that I am not thinking about you, because I obviously am as I am writing in my diary.

The mundane normality and stress of things is healing and distracting.

Thank goodness.

I will write again later when my sanity returns.

10.17 p.m.

It never returned!!

21 August 2009
10.41 p.m.

Exactly one month since that call; it has been a blur.

Back from work about 10.00 p.m. and have spent the last forty minutes calming down!

My mum phoned me at work to tell me that Audrey had been on to Cheryl questioning why I was coming to see you. You are too ill and are wondering why everyone is visiting you.

I am confused.

You know you have cancer, and that it is serious.

You are a grown man.

We have had conversations about the fact that loved ones want to see you because cancer is a scary word.

Audrey also questioned why Nathan was coming to see you when he hasn't bothered with you for years.

Let's just get this straight. Your nineteen-year-old grandson wants to see you. You haven't seen him for years because you chose to maintain a difficult relationship with your daughter and punish her children also. Your wife has poisoned your thoughts on as many of your family as she could manage whilst trying to convince everyone in a sickly sweet way that she hasn't. For what reason I will never know.

Why you could never see it, I will never know. Then there are times when I have looked into your eyes, and I think you could see it, but you had made your bed!

Why does that woman not just allow the people who love you dearly to grieve?

Why does she need to have control and take every opportunity to stick the knife in?

Wicked! Wicked! Wicked!

I will be down to see you, and I will be bringing Nathan and Caroline.

It may be the last time I see you. Would you deny me that?

I would walk over hot coals to see you as often as I can before you die.

What right has she got to try and take that away from me?

I was talking to Janice about it tonight. Did you know that when you stayed at Janice's that time, within five minutes of meeting her Audrey was slagging all your family off including me except Shaun and Rebecca?

What sort of person does that?

No wonder your opinions have been so negative.

She could not taint your love for me though could she.

I could do no wrong, and there is a depth to our relationship that she will never, never understand.

The love of a father for his firstborn daughter and the love of a daughter for her dad.

That bond will not be broken even by death.

Anyway, I will be down to see you again next week, like it or not.

I will sit with you, hold your hand, and talk to you.

And once again, for you, I will be polite and nice to Audrey.

I will have reframed my anger and disgust and be the better person, like I have done for the last thirteen years.

Goodnight, Dad.

Please wake up with the morning light.

Remember when we used to go to Blackpool at the weekends? We would sing about hot doughnuts and hot meat pies all the way home. You would wear all the daft hats, go on all the rides, and act the clown all day. So much laughter, and so many happy memories. But I could have gone to the end of the road with you, Dad, and had as much fun; you were hilarious.

To understand your parents' love, you must raise children yourself.
Chinese proverb

22 August 2009
9.15 a.m.

I am calm.

A few hours sleep and the kids around me, and the anger has melted away.

I still think the behaviour that Audrey is showing at the minute is unforgivable. However, I am prepared to stand up to this challenge, be mature and calm, and show her the way to behave.

I would do anything for you.

She would probably be surprised to know that Shaun is totally disgusted with the way she is behaving and the unnecessary hurt she is causing me, and he really does not want to see her again after you are gone.

I am not sure I can do that to my kids, they love her as "nannie" and know none of this, and it would not be fair.

3.33 p.m.

Lots of talks today.

Auntie Cheryl, my mum, Audrey.

Mum understands how hard this is for me at the minute. She fully supports me and despises Audrey for what she is doing.

I have thought things through all day, and I am prepared to forgive and compromise to keep the peace for you.

I am prepared to lie, be nice, bite my lip, smile, and vent after I leave.

I am prepared to accept whatever you want when I come to see you: if you don't want to see the kids then that is fine; if you can't talk to me then that's fine; if you are in bed then that is also fine.

I have booked a hotel just around the corner from where you live so I can be there in five minutes if needs be.

I don't want anything other than to see you and say my goodbyes in my own way. They won't be verbal as that would not be fair on you, but mentally I need to do what I need to do.

I have reconciled that you may not make it to my next visit with me going into hospital on 10th September.

I have already accepted that your death is out of my control and also in Audrey's.

I am not angry at you or at cancer because we all have to die.

I am not going to allow that negative feeling of anger back into my emotions now. I am going to focus on gratitude, forgiveness, and love because the anger is making me behave badly towards the ones I love.

Audrey is playing the martyr well as she has done as long as I have known her. She is physically and emotionally drained, and it is hard work (her words). But she wants to do it. I can empathise. I will say the right things to make her feel better, and I will ignore the festering feeling in the pit of my stomach.

I WILL NOT allow anger to consume me and let my beloved family suffer.

I am going to fake it and be positive, and hopefully in faking it the false positives will become real.

I will listen sweetly on the phone and agree about the hard time she is having and say how sorry I am.

I will give her a hug when I come down and hold her hand too.

I will do whatever she asks of me and show not one glimmer of anger or resentment.

I will do all of this for you, because you chose to be with her, and you love her, so there has to be some good somewhere.

I genuinely think that she does not know how destructive she is with her criticism of all and sundry, and I would put a million pound on the fact that she is not aware of her flaws and what people really think of her because of them.

To be that far away from having empathy for and truly understanding others without judgement must be an uncomfortable place to be all of the time.

I really dislike the emotional feelings of hate, resentment, and envy; they don't make you feel good.

To live with those feelings all of the time and not be able to find forgiveness or gratitude must be debilitating for her. She seems to live in an imaginary world where she is never wrong, yet lacks so many life experiences to have had enough points of reference to be right about people.

Quite sad really.

But why would I waste any of my time and energy on somebody that I do not really care about.

It is you I care about, and that is why I am writing this diary.

I hope that in writing this I can achieve two goals: to raise money for cancer research, to connect to others and help them with their emotions.

I hope I can go some way to doing that for you.

Well, I must go and get ready for work again. I will not write again tonight because I really do need to try and get some sleep when I come in.

I also need to spend a bit of time with Shaun; he has been a bit neglected of late.

As far as men go, there has only ever been you and him. The others were just learnings, allowing me to appreciate a wonderful dad and a wonderful husband.

How people treat you is their karma; how you react is yours.
Wayne Dyer

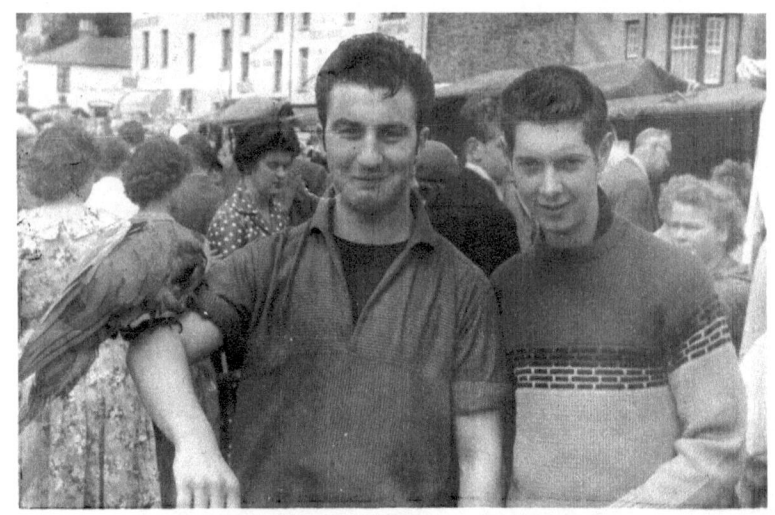

My dad as a teenager, with parrot!

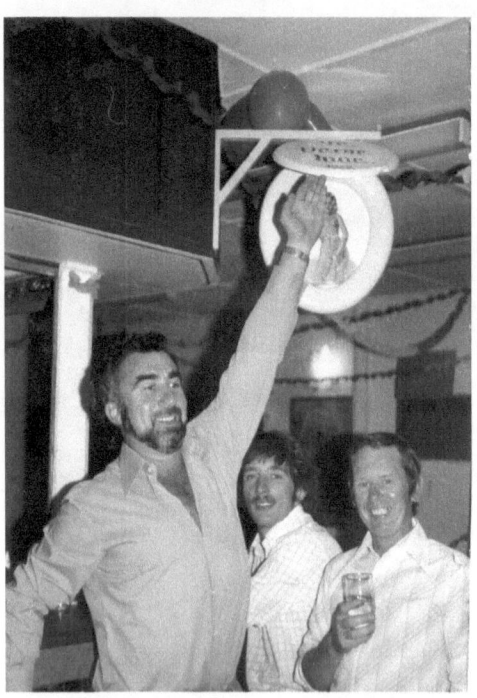

Having fun in Indonesia with his work colleagues; how I remember him.

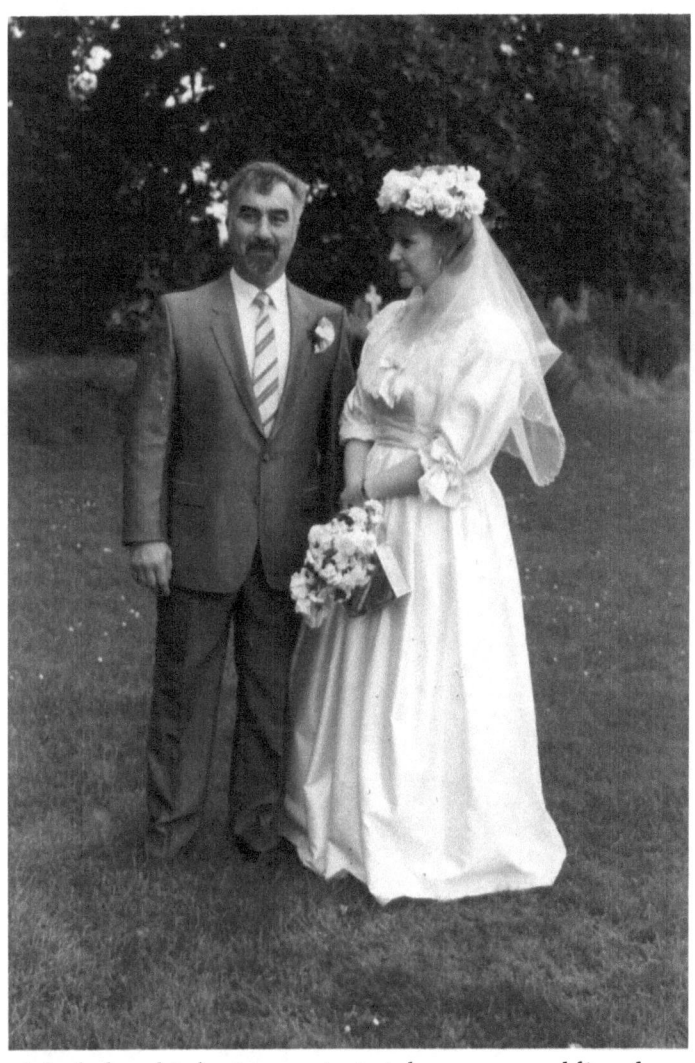

My dad and I sharing a private joke on my wedding day.

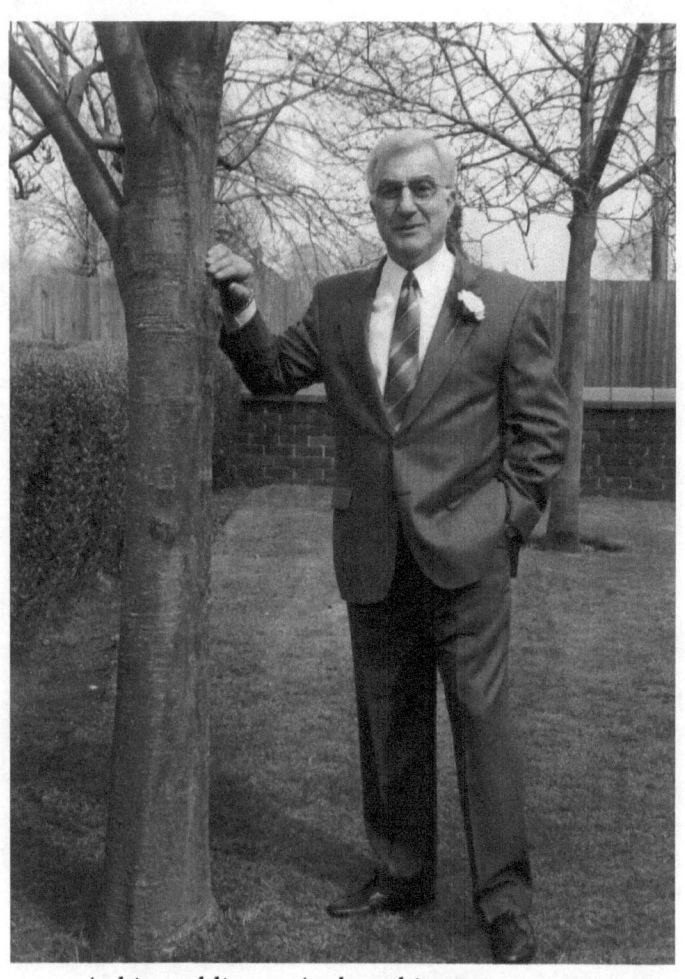

At his wedding to Audrey thirteen years ago.

23 August 2009
8.46 p.m.

Been to work; same old day.

Called at Amanda's on the way home again and had a cuppa.

I asked her to paint a card for you last time I saw her, and she has done it. It is beautiful.

I have just written the verse to go in it, a valuable piece from two ladies who will be very famous one day!

I hope that you can understand the message and that I am the last person to send you a card because I have struggled to find a reason when my dad is dying!

My card is my farewell, just in case this is the last time I see you.

They don't make cards that have that message.

For my dad..........
For all the times you said there, there
For everything you've done
For all the times you showed you care
I am grateful for every one

You taught me well, you are the best
Here's something you should know
You stand head and shoulders above the rest
My dad, my friend, my HERO!

Now you are ill, it's hard to bear
For those so far away
I think about you constantly
And, I love you, is all I can say

So thank you dad for the lessons learned
You said little but I knew
Love and respect are definitely earned
And if anyone earned them, it is you

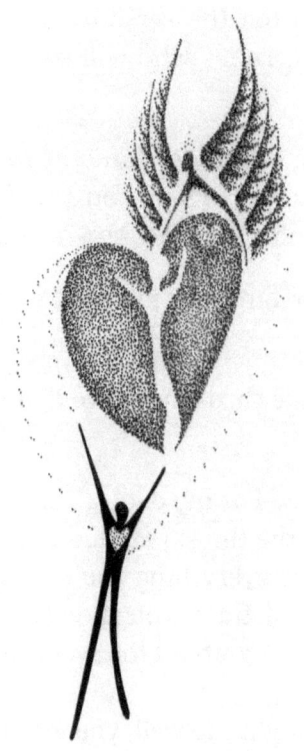

Farewell. Illustration by Amanda Hall Younger

I find my mind constantly wandering to that dark-haired, Arab-looking man that brought me up and dreading seeing the shadow of a man that is awaiting me on my pending visit.

After talking to Amanda today I am actually angry at the system, that is, the National Health Service.

You have remarried, so Audrey is your next of kin.

She is the one who will receive the twenty-four-hour telephone support and counselling when she needs it.

She is the one who will sit with you next week and hear your prognosis.

And she is the one, if you are not able, who will make the decision about your treatment.

What about your two daughters?

Where do we fit in?

We love you just as much.

Audrey will be with you when you leave this earth, and I am completely reliant on her having the courtesy to phone me in time to make the four- hour drive.

It all feels so wrong.

I think they should look at the procedures and include children in the communication and support system, particularly when there is remarriage.

I feel so helpless, lost, and distant, at a time when I want to feel close.

I may look into and challenge the system at some point when I feel stronger.

I really do feel calmer today; maybe I had to go through the anger in order to get it out of my system.

I am sure that Mr Anger and I will meet again yet! However, we have currently parted company, and Mr Calm is here.

I will always remember your first visit after my daughter Rebecca was born. The way you looked at her was a treasure; locked away in my memory for the rest of my days. I imagine that it was the way you looked at me when I was born, for you have looked at me that way many times. There were real tears of pride and joy in your eyes, and an acknowledgement that I had done good. Thank you for those moments; nobody can ever own them but me.

How pleasant it is for a father to sit at his child's board. It is like an aged man reclining under the shadow of an oak which he has planted.
Walter Scott

Night, night.

Sleep tight.

Please wake up with the morning light.

24 August 2009
6.56 p.m.

I am coming to see you tomorrow, and I am filled with trepidation.

I hope that I can be strong for you.

Nathan is coming with me, and I am meeting Caroline.

The kids are staying at home with my mum. You can't cope, so I reflected and decided to leave them here.

I am shattered from work today and feel mentally drained from lack of sleep, but nothing will stop me coming to see you.

I have just had a text message from Audrey saying you are really ill and she is emotionally and physically drained.

I really do feel for her and want to be of some support.

I am torn between anger, empathy, and sympathy!

I don't feel angry today but still feel angry at Audrey for her sheer lack of interest and understanding; then in the next thought I feel sorry that she has to go through this.

There are things about her that I like and I can tolerate; like I said before, you love her, so she can't be all bad. It is simply her inability to forgive and be grateful for people. She harbours too much bitterness and replays it like a stuck record, convincing herself and others that her version is the only version.

There is never a thought about what the other person feels or thinks; they are a certain way and that is it, end of story.

In her world people can't change, grow, learn, or be sorry for their behaviour. If only she knew how narrow minded and destructive that thought process is!

I am sure that she is completely convincing and that all of her friends think she is wonderful and I am the wicked stepdaughter. She is great at telling the sob story.

Never mind; that is how it is, and only she can change that if she wants too.

I like to observe the bad behaviour in others and correct my own behaviour accordingly.

The ability to learn and grow is empowering; it makes you strong, forgiving, and open. I am happy as I am.

Well, tonight I have talked to Viv, Sheena (who have now reconnected because of you!), Ange, and Janice.

My life is full of people who are grateful for my opinion, and I take that as a compliment.

Just wish that I could have that hour-long conversation with the one person that I want to have it with at the minute, you!

That is what I will miss the most, being able to talk to you.

I promise I still will, and I will look for the signs.

See you tomorrow, Dad.

Night, night.

Sleep tight.

Please wake up with the morning light.

I remember when Billy and I split up and how nasty it all was. I have never seen you so defensive of me and so angry with another human being. In fact, I just can't remember you angry other than that. Wow, what an achievement that is; my kids won't be able to say that about me – although now I have recognised that, I will try harder. What helped me the most during that time were our talks and you just being there. I am sure I talked far more than you, and you just listened to me vent, but it meant a lot. You were there for all the important bits, Dad. I am big enough to deal with it on my own now; this year has taught me that. What bigger hurt will I ever have to face than losing a beloved parent? I can do anything now.

Listening is a magnetic and strange thing, a creative force. The friends who listen to us are the ones we move toward. When we are listened to, it creates us, makes us unfold and expand.
Author unknown

27 August 2009
2.15 p.m.

Nathan and I arrived yesterday at around 2.30 p.m. and checked into a hotel. I called Audrey to tell her we had arrived, and we came straight round to see you.

Audrey was distraught. She had her friend Beryl with her, and she had obviously suffered since the last time I saw her – thin and drawn.

We chatted for a while, and Audrey's tears were impossible for her to control; she cried a river, sobbing and asking why.

We came upstairs to see you; initially Audrey would not leave us alone with you, but eventually she left the room after about five minutes.

You knew it was me.

Your face softened as I held your hand and told you that I loved you.

You were at home where you wanted to be, but you looked so much worse than the last time I saw you in hospital.

You looked like a dying man.

You could not keep your eyes open and could hardly speak.

But you knew it was me.

I had no more than ten minutes with you.

Nathan was shocked and really upset by what he saw; that big, powerful man was no more.

You asked us if we had come to give you your last rites and crossed your chest; this took both mine and Nathan's breath away.

I told you not to be so daft. I hadn't been to church since I was christened. Audrey was back in the room at that point and corrected me, reminding me that I had been in church for your wedding to her and my children's christenings.

Sorry for being inaccurate!

A bit distracted.

We came back downstairs and stayed for a couple of hours to talk to Audrey.

Nathan was visibly distressed and had to compose himself before coming into the living room.

Audrey then talked about her pain through her tears.

My heart went out to her; however, she made absolutely sure she emphasised some specific things:

"Brian does not want to leave ME" – four times.

"He is worried about how I will cope on my own."

"He asked for his will the other day."

For the record, I have absolutely no interest in the will unless there are personal items you want me or the kids to have.

I look after myself, make my own wealth, and I neither want nor need your money if there is any (which I am pretty sure there is not).

Why she even had to bring that up, I do not know, unless it is to broach the subject now so that I won't say anything later.

Well, it does not matter to me.

You are all that matters to me.

She can have everything. I have memories that can never be hers – precious and treasured.

Audrey then informed me that you did not want to see Caroline. She was on her way, so I texted her and diverted her to our hotel. We left approximately ten minutes after that and met Caroline.

We had a wonderful night with Caz, catching up on what we had missed. You would really love her, Dad. She is like me but even more beautiful. A strong lady who knows what she wants.

In placing yourself completely in Audrey and Derek's lives and cutting out your family, you have missed out on some fantastic people.

I will make up for that for you.

I will champion communication and love, because I

must learn from your errors. I respect your choices; they were yours. That does not mean I have to agree with them. Neither do I 100 per cent believe that it is what you really felt in your heart.

I will only know that when we meet again on the other side.

I am writing this entry in the waiting room of accident and emergency at Wigan hospital having followed the ambulance in.

Audrey texted me at 10.30 this morning to say that you were worse and that she was bringing the doctor in. We came straight over. She was very upset and explained how bad things had been. She looked terrible, not well, and very tired.

She told us that they were going to bring you into Wigan by ambulance, but she was reluctant to let you go.

I can understand that.

We sat and waited for the ambulance, and here I am trying to do something to distract me from breaking down in front of all and sundry.

You looked so ill when I peered through the doors of the assessment area. Oh my God, Dad, I don't want you to go!

So here I am; waiting, waiting, waiting, and waiting for bad news.

Ange is on her way on the train. I phoned her and

told her to come, just in case. I have to pick her up at the station at 6.30 p.m.

My dad ... you spent your life being my provider, protector, supporter, adviser. Now all I can hope for is that you become my guardian angel.

Grief is bad.

Cancer is worse.

Cancer, eating away at you, taking you so quickly from those that love you so much.

I will do anything that I have to do now to have this diary published. I want to raise as much money as possible for cancer research. There has to be a way that a more proactive approach can be available for my kids. And if I have to suffer it too, I pray for euthanasia to be legal in this country so that I don't have to go like you.

People have said to me, "Thank goodness it was quick." Well, it has not felt "quick" to me. It has felt like a daily roller-coaster of hope and despair, tugging at your pain centre and making everything hurt.

Waiting, waiting, waiting.

Audrey keeps coming out to see us and give us an update on your ramblings – like that makes me feel better.

However, I recognise that is her way of coping with the situation.

I can find forgiveness, you know.

The hurt I have felt at Audrey and Derek's behaviour will pass. I am capable of forgiveness and gratitude.

I will never be able to thank Audrey enough for the enjoyment and happiness she gave you over the last thirteen years. It is the one thing that allows me to overlook the negative behaviour and bitterness that is demonstrated verbally each time we meet.

She asked Nathan if he had regrets today about not making more of an effort to see you over the last few years. Of course he has! But whose fault was it?

Everyone's except his; he was a child caught up in silly adult arguments.

Anyway this is not a time for blame or regret.

Thank you, Audrey, for all you did for my beloved dad; everything else is just words.

If you blame others for your failures, do you credit them with your success?

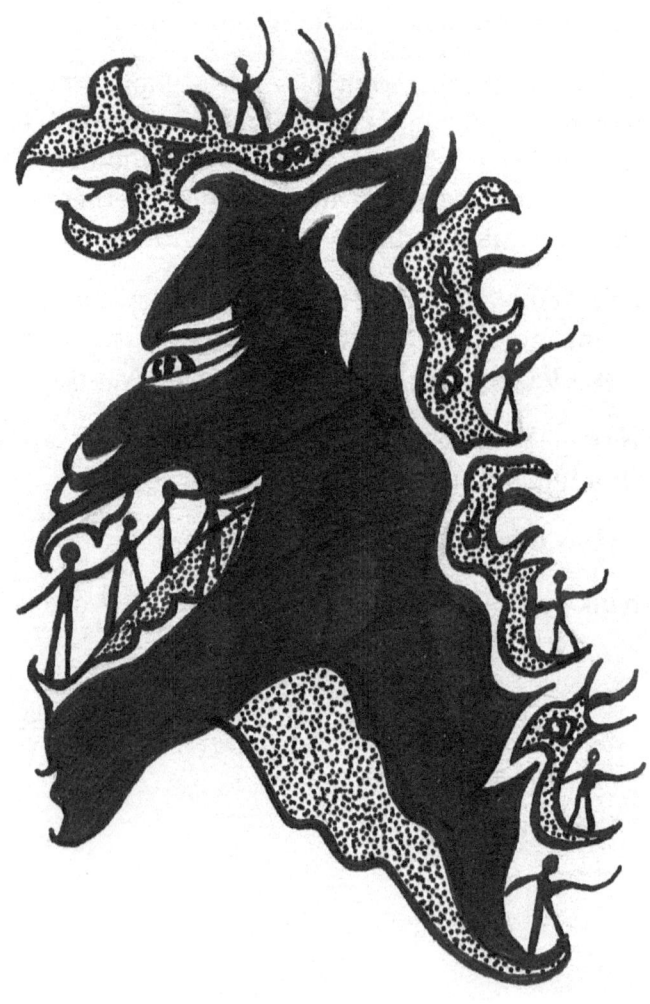

Cancer Monster. Illustration by Amanda Hall Younger

10.55 p.m.

Well, we left Audrey at about 9.45 p.m. after having a drink and a chat with her. Had a few drinks in the bar.

I have now lost the opportunity to read out your eulogy because apparently you made a comment about not wanting any of that nonsense at your funeral after attending somebody else's.

Was that another of those defence mechanisms?

Was it bold and tough boy talk with Derek?

Or did you really mean it?

I will never know. But Audrey says you don't want it, and her word is gospel.

So, Dad, the one tribute I could make to you in front of family and friends has been taken. If you really knew me, Audrey too, you would know for sure that I would not write soppy mush. You would also know I would practice with professional flair. I would keep tears at bay, the message short and to the point showing respect and acknowledgement.

But yet another thing was taken away by Audrey in her inability to see the opinion of others.

I am not going to dwell on it. The last entry in this diary will be on the day of your funeral, and I will close with your eulogy.

My tribute to you will be heard by far more than the attendees of your funeral.

I am just accepting every shove further away as it comes now.

I can be hurt no more.

27 August 2009
6.42 a.m.

THE POWER OF WORDS

I woke up at 6.15 this morning in the hotel room with Ange and Nathan; I couldn't sleep.

I woke up with the power of words in my head.

Words have the power to cut and bleed, to hurt like a knife wound deep in your gut.

They also have the power to heal, to empower, and to feed the soul.

How you choose to use words is a reflection of your emotional intelligence and ability to truly connect to others.

Some people use words without considering the impact they may have on the recipient.

To know the impact of what you say and how you say it is great knowledge indeed.

Why did I wake up with that on my mind?

You could be abrupt, cutting at times, and you could dismiss people as meaningless to you. I truly believe this was a mixture of honesty and defence mechanisms to protect you from hurt or from showing your true feelings. I believe that this sent mixed messages to those around you in that sometimes, when you were using a defence mechanism, it could be interpreted as you dismissing a person as meaningless.

For example, Ange. You said you didn't care, yet your eyes told a different story. I could see what you felt; you were different with me.

Then there is Audrey. She wears her heart on her sleeve and overexpresses. I observed her closely yesterday because I spent the day with her.

In expressing her feelings, she often says hurtful things without even knowing it. When she talks about her pain, it appears that she has no empathy and comprehension of anyone else's; this, in itself, can be hurtful.

But, on close observation yesterday, I have come to the conclusion that there is no malice intended. She is trying to express herself in the only way she knows. I have vented many times in this diary about her bad behaviour, and I don't take it back because that is the impact it can have, and has had over the years.

However, I think that I reached a new level of understanding and tolerance yesterday.

She was just so frail and hurt by the thought of losing you. For you to have been loved so much by anyone other than Ange and me is a great comfort to me.

I am at peace.

People say life is too short all of the time, but few do anything different after saying it.

I am going to do, Dad.

I am going to live every minute and do everything in my power to bring others together.

I am a teacher, a philosopher, a conduit for great communication, and a giver.

Watch over me with a smile, Dad.

11.03 p.m.

We begged the nurses to let us come in and see you one last time today before driving home, and they said yes.

You were very poorly, and it was a hard goodbye.

I have accepted that I may never see you alive again, and that I may have no influence or input into your funeral.

That does not mean that I am not in pain.

Yet again your face is a strong image in my head, and I can't sleep.

I love you so much, Dad.

I have been to my introduction meeting with the Samaritans this evening.

I am so keen to volunteer. I think it will be really rewarding and that I will learn a lot.

I have not been very nice to Shaun since I arrived home, but we have time to patch that up. I couldn't help myself. I just feel drained and tired.

I have my pre-op assessment at Ashington tomorrow. I wish I didn't have to go for the operation. I am scared you will die while I am in, and I will miss the opportunity to get to you.

Never mind. What will be will be.

Although I am so, so sad, I am feeling positive about my life and future. I have no doubts about my success and that all will be good.

I can pretty much face anything after this year, and if I can remain forward-thinking and positive, through this, then I can get through anything.

You will be so proud of me; you can tell me when we meet again.

Night, night.

Sleep tight.

I pray for you to pass peacefully in your sleep tonight.

I asked grandads Jack and George to meet you; they sent a sign. I believe that you will be met with the open arms of loving souls, and I will expect your open arms at my own time of passing. Good men deserve a good greeting, and you were always a good man.

As a well-spent day brings happy sleep, so life well used brings happy death.
Leonardo da Vinci

28 August 2009
10.49 p.m.

Well, I have had the call from Audrey to tell me you are dying.

The cancer is in your brain and blood, and you have deteriorated fast.

Audrey is distraught.

I feel helpless.

You will leave me tonight, maybe tomorrow, definitely soon.

Although I have been preparing myself, I am numb again.

For the first time, I can't cry.

Initially I did when I came off the phone to Audrey, but now I can't.

I don't know what to feel.

She said you were in pain; the doctors were coming to medicate you.

I don't want you to be in pain.

Please, God, take him quickly so that he does not suffer.

I can't bear the thought of you suffering.

Please take him now, in his sleep, and let him rest in peace.

Here come the tears...

And gone just as quick!!

Audrey sounded in so much pain. I genuinely wish I could give her a hug.

Who would believe that you and I walked the dogs together for a good mile in April?

Only four months ago, you were fine.

Or so you led us all to believe.

You were complaining about your sore legs, and I suspect that there was more and for much longer.

That was our last dad-daughter talk. Our private time between only you and me.

Nobody else was privy to those conversations. I will treasure that particular one for the rest of my days, and only you and I will know what was said.

You came alive when we spent time alone together.

I need you to let me know you are OK.

Send me a sign.

I don't want to stop this entry because my next one may be about your death.

Very final.

I don't know what I will write then, as emotions keep taking me by surprise.

I am now eating chocolate, to try and make me feel better, at 11 o'clock at night!! I know I will suffer, but at least I won't have a hangover.

I am stuck for words; I am going to bed.

I am dreading the call.

I wanted a perfect ending. Now I've learned, the hard way, that some poems don't rhyme, and some stories don't have a clear beginning, middle, and end. Life is about not knowing, having to change, taking the moment and making the best of it, without knowing what's going to happen next. Delicious Ambiguity.
Gilda Radner

29 August 2009
8.11 p.m.

Still no phone call.

Just a text from Audrey at 11.23 a.m. to say you were still the same, sedated on morphine and asleep.

At least that means no pain.

The morphine may keep you breathing and alive for longer, but it won't change the facts and the inevitable conclusion.

Ange has had a really bad day.

I have been to work and got on with my day, but it is torture not knowing when the phone call will come.

Whilst the call does not come, I can pretend all is normal until the moment, memory, or reminder arrives to stop me and force out a tear.

Shake your head, take a deep breath, and get on with it!

I need you to be at peace now so that everyone can move on.

You really wouldn't allow an animal to continue in pain.

Yet we postpone death with drugs in the people we love dearly, why?

I have to say that watching you die has given me the clarity to make a very important decision.

I will not go like that.

The image of you in the hospital on Thursday before we came home will haunt me for the rest of my life.

I couldn't write about it on Thursday because I was so angry and distressed. I actually think I suppressed it in order to be strong for Ange and Nathan.

When the nurses agreed to let us in to see you before we travelled home, Ange, Nathan, and I waltzed in with an electric fan and a six pack of lucozade. You had been hot and thirsty the night before.

As we walked towards your bed, the curtains were half shut, and you were sitting on a wheelchair, teetering on the front edge with your boxers round your knees.

As we moved closer and could see properly, you had obviously had a wee in a bottle and had the bottle in your hand. You had underpants on, and there was a sticker hanging out of the back saying, "I am clean." Both Ange and I went into autopilot moved you onto the bed, pulled your boxers up, and removed the bottle. None of the nurses were showing any interest; you seemed to have been abandoned.

You are a proud man, so you would have been embarrassed if you had had the strength of mind and body.

WHAT ABOUT DIGNITY!!!!!!

Bloody angry irate – so much so I have just shut down for two days and been unable to make sense of it.

My poor, lovely dad.

How dare they not care for you!

How dare they treat you like that!

How dare God take you away!

I have asked Shaun to make sure that if I go first, then he will take me to Dignitas. I will not end my life like you have.

We are going to have our wills done once you are at peace. There will be no room for second guessing – they will be specific and directive.

Forty days since you were diagnosed, and I sit here waiting for you to die.

I can do nothing of any substance. I just don't seem to have the ability today.

Normally I am thinking, being creative, working, and enjoying the kids – all out the window.

I am just existing and checking the phone.

9.09 p.m.

Text from Audrey – no change.

I remember in one of our "put the world to rights" conversations, you saying to me that you were deeply in love with your two little girls until they became teenagers and wanted to change the world. I think that you really struggled with me being so strong-willed and independent, and I distinctly remember Ange being your favourite because she was still "little." I never had a problem with that because I have always had the self-confidence and never needed anyone's approval. What I know for sure is that we found that closeness again in the last ten years and that you have been a good friend and confidant. I know that I surpassed your expectations and that you really love me and are proud of me. You never had to say a word because your eyes told such a story. Thank you for being you and being in my life; you made a difference. I will see you every morning when I look in the mirror, and I know I am like you – so you will live on in me.

The secret of health for both mind and body is not to mourn for the past, worry about the future, or anticipate troubles but to live in the present moment wisely and earnestly.
Buddha

30 August 2009
9.23 p.m.

Still no call, so you are still with us and still sedated.

I have had to bring back some normality, so I have been to the pictures with Shaun and the kids and out for a meal.

I had to switch the phone off and was worried all through the film that I would get a call from Audrey and miss it.

I have just sent a text to Audrey asking for an update as I have heard nothing since last night.

It is so hard not being there for you, not knowing how you are hour by hour; you are all I think about.

I am doing OK at the moment, holding it together well.

I spoke to Hilary for an hour today. I enjoyed every minute, so pleased I have her back. She did a very special thing – reminded me who I am. She may not even have realised it, but she did. I have been accepting of Audrey's comments about you not wanting an eulogy, and, in doing so, I have behaved like you and not me – anything for an easy life! Amanda King – not fight and be outspoken – I don't think so! I will try my best without behaving badly to pay that tribute to my dad. Thanks, Auntie Hils. You are a star!

Come on, Audrey, text me an update. I am restless and need to know.

She is probably holding your hand while you are dying, while I am two hundred miles away wondering.

Well, I am only your daughter!

I am going to watch some TV to distract myself, and I hope that I get a text so that I can sleep tonight.

Stepmothers – they marry the man you love and try to make him their own. Men are so fickle that they declare their undying love to this new woman, never considering the daughter who will never fall out of love with them. You can't go down the pub, play golf, watch football, or slap each other on the back and have a manly relationship. Between a dad and his daughter is a special, loving relationship containing real emotion and hero worship. A complicated and highly charged environment to place yourself in the middle of, yet so many women do and are surprised by the resentment. Stepmothers, if your man has a daughter, there will always be another woman with whom you cannot compete; brace yourself!

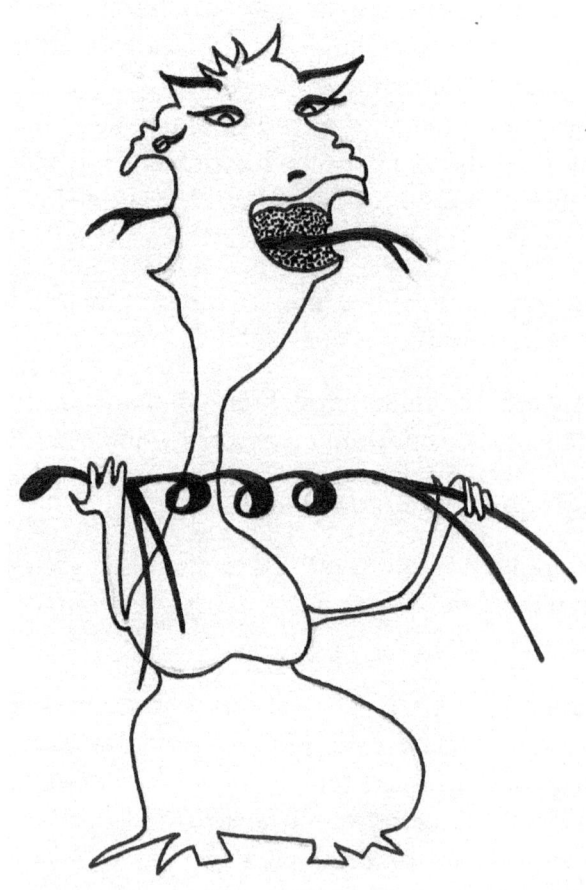

Stepmonsters. Illustarted by Amanda Hall Younger

10.02 p.m.

Text from Audrey: "He is very poorly. He wants to come home to his own bed – and me! Will text tomorrow when I can dry my tears."

Sometimes there are no words.

Sometimes there are no quotes or memories.

Sometimes it is just the end of a very hard day.

Sometimes there is only emptiness.

31 August 2009
2.19 p.m.

I will be writing this piece on and off all day as there is a lot on my mind; so be prepared!

Death: a subject for discussion.

It appears that everyone has an opinion on death, as in what is appropriate and what is not.

What I should do with your eulogy, how I should behave, if I should speak to Audrey or not... yada, yada.

So I would like to state my wishes.

I would then like to outline in finite detail what I want to happen when my time comes so that my children do not have to listen to anyone else's opinion.

What I want:

I would really like to read the eulogy out at your funeral, because I would like to deliver a tribute to you, simple as that. I do not need or want control. I do not want to choose hymns or music. I do not want to invite anyone.

I just want to turn up with my family, read a tribute to you in front of family and friends, say goodbye, and go.

I am OK with Audrey having control; I want no fallouts, arguments, or anything else.

But, apparently, I can't have that because you made a comment one day, and Audrey can't find it in her heart to allow me to have any sort of healing or farewell unless under her complete control.

I am going to discuss that with the vicar once I know where the funeral is, and I will listen to his advice.

My thoughts when it is my turn are as follows:
This is my message to Rebecca and Daniel, my beloved children. Firstly I want you both to know that I love you both equally and more than I can even begin to describe to you as there are no appropriate words.
I will love you always no matter what you do or how many mistakes you make, even if you become an axe wielding, homicidal maniac – you will still be my axe wielding homicidal maniac!
There has never been a day, neither will there ever be a day when I am not filled with wonder and pride over your achievements, no matter how small.
Your dad and I created you out of love, and love is

what we have for you every day of your lives and beyond.

When it is my time to go, I ask of you only one thing: play "Stairway to Heaven" by Led Zeppelin at my funeral.

Other than that, I am completely cool with whatever you want to do. You can bury me, cremate me, scatter me; it does not matter a bit as I won't be there and I don't care.

You can read one or a hundred eulogies; you can dance, sing, cry, and laugh, whatever you want, as long as it brings you closure and healing.

I will accept anything from you; in fact, I will love whatever you do because it is you.

Don't be frightened to decide. Do not be afraid that you will offend, because I will be perched on a cloud somewhere smiling and saying, "That's my kids. Aren't they great?"

What does it matter what is said or done? Once you are dead, if it brings healing for others, surely that is the main point.

Isn't a funeral meant to be a last goodbye? Then say goodbye your way!

I will not dictate to you in life. I will empower you to make your own decisions and stand by them, learn from them, and be proud of them – even if they are ridiculous; so why would I dictate to you in death?

My song request is just that; consider yourselves DJs playing the last track of the night!

You are both great, beautiful, clever people who have made my life worth living, every single minute of it; so celebrate that achievement.

Celebrate my life because I lived it to the full every day.

I have no regrets or what ifs; I just did it all. If I can say that now, at forty-four, then take my word for it, by the time the end comes, if you are not embarrassed by me and proud of me at the same time, then I will be very surprised.

You have my permission to do what the hell you want and have a ball. Don't be sad. Be strong like I have taught you.

I am writing this diary to your grandad, but for you because life is learning and sometimes we forget to pass it on. How many parents can say they shared such a learning with their children? Whatever the number, I wish it were more.

My only other request, nay, demand, is that I die with dignity. Do not hold onto the body for your own benefit. I wish to go of my own accord, in Switzerland if necessary, with a simple drink or pill. Do not be afraid because I am not. I will not go at the hands of the NHS treated with less dignity than a dying animal.

Anyway, Dad, now you know how I feel.

You being diagnosed with this awful disease and dying so quickly have taught me so much.

I find myself looking for learning every day and have to admit I have learnt something from every single human interaction in my life.

This is just one of this year's many learning opportunities.

I know you are going to a better place.

In fact, I just spoke with Lou, and that is exactly what she said.

How lucky am I to have such great people in my life; I treasure them all.

Being alive means you have a duty.

A duty to live it and enjoy it.

You did what you wanted to do, and I will do what I want to do.

We will both have learned what we were meant to.

9.07 p.m.

Call from Audrey. You have gone into a coma, and they do not expect you to last the night, maximum a couple of days.

I think I will sign off with that thought and pray that you go peacefully tonight; it is your time.

Goodnight, Dad.

Sleep tight.

Please make your final journey tonight.

Beth could not reason upon or explain the faith that gave her courage and patience to give up life, and cheerfully wait for death. Like a confiding child, she asked no questions, but left everything to God and

nature, Father and Mother of us all, feeling sure that
they, and they only, could teach and strengthen heart
and spirit for this life and the life to come.
Louisa May Alcott, *Little Women*, chapter 36

1 September 2009
4.23 p.m.

You died today at around lunchtime; don't know the exact time as the call from Audrey was short, but that is irrelevant.

Audrey did not make it on time to be with you; why she was not with you every second until you went, I do not know and do not want to know.

You died alone, and she will have to live with that. I would have been there if I had not been made to feel so unwelcome.

Forty-three days ago, I started this diary because I wanted to document the real emotion, real issues, and real occurrences on a cancer journey so that it may help others.

Who knew it would be such a short journey with so much emotion and so many issues and occurrences?

I have spent all afternoon phoning people to let them know and trying to control my own emotion.

I have told the kids. Becca very, very upset; Dan asked if you had gone to heaven.

I said yes, and he said, "That is OK. Then we will see him again." Sometimes I wish you could just bottle the comments of children; they are so wise.

As for me, well, I have been preparing myself, and I will control it like you would have.

I will have my moments, I am sure, but I said goodbye to you last week.

I have been forced into an early goodbye because of the situation with Audrey and her need to own you.

I am at peace with that, and I just hope and pray that you are at peace also.

Please forgive me for the bad thoughts about Audrey. I have tried so hard for years now to compromise and make it right for you. I think I did a pretty good job actually, but she was cruel with words, turned you into something that I know you are not, and encouraged you to cut people out of your life that should have been part of it.

It is almost like she wanted to erase your past and make your time with her the only thing that mattered.

Well, I loved you despite that, unconditionally. No judgement, no neediness, no control; just pure, unconditional love.

Thank you for loving me back.

You gave me the gift of being here for forty-four years and eleven months of my growing time. It is safe to leave me now as I will manage on my own. Thank you for that time; I am a better person because of it. I will look after Ange and all of your grandchildren for you, trust me.

I need to prepare myself now for my interview with the Samaritans tonight because I really want to do this.

I will write again later, Dad. I love you, and I will miss you.

Father! - to God himself we cannot give a holier name. William Wordsworth

9.26 p.m.

Back from my interview; think it went well. I am even keener to get involved now.

Amanda gave me a book today: *Embraced by the Light – what happens when you die,* by Betty J. Eadie. I started reading it earlier, and it is helping to keep me feeling positive. I think I may need to stay up and finish it tonight.

I was at Amanda's when I received the call from Audrey. I think I was meant to be there so that I could cope better. She has had as much of an impact in my life as I have had in hers. Some people are just meant to meet at a certain time; it's part of the learning. I see us having a long association and friendship. I love her creativity.

I feel so at peace for you, and I have been able to keep the tears at bay all day. Just a few near misses, but, all in all, I think you would be proud of how I have held it together.

Shaun got the brunt of it as usual. Poor him, he always gets it. Part of the job description, I am afraid.

Good job he loves me; I am grateful for that.

Becca was upset tonight when I arrived back. She told me that she had said a prayer for you and seen a flock of birds pass, which was a sign from you. She is a smart girl, you know, way ahead of her years. Bit like me, really.

Anyway, Dad, I will keep talking to you now until your funeral. As you know, I really want to read the eulogy for you. You need to trust me that I will not go sloppy and slushy. Once the funeral is over, I will add your eulogy as the final entry in this diary and close a chapter in my life. I can then hold you in my thoughts and my heart until we are reunited again. I will draw strength from you and try to always make you proud.

I loved you in life, I love you no less in death. In fact death has taken our relationship to a whole new level; I can talk and you will always listen, distance is no longer an issue.
Mandy King

Becca and Dan have been saying this for you every night:

I see the moon and the moon sees me;

God bless grandad and God bless me.

God bless you, Dad. I will sleep well tonight, knowing you are no longer in pain and that you are in heaven!

2 September 2009
5.37 p.m.

I seem to have spent half the day on the phone. Mum called this morning. She is really upset – which I did not really expect and I found very emotional. She is coming to the funeral, though, which I am delighted about. Viv called because she is struggling with her current work situation and wanted advice. She felt bad for calling me, but I was pleased as it allowed me to talk about something else for a change.

I called Ange to check on her. She is still very upset, driven by guilt. I have asked her to forgive herself and try and get on with life – easier said than done for some people, though.

Caroline phoned me to see how I was, and we had a chat.

I am OK.

I am surprisingly OK.

I have felt a bit lazy today. Haven't done very much. A bit listless, but emotionally OK.

I finished the book I started, and it has really given me something to consider and research. My gut feeling: it is a revelation, yet it is not. I feel like I already knew. However, I still wanted to know; it sounds a bit crazy, but that is the only way I can describe it.

I would advise anyone struggling with grief to get hold of a copy and read it; it only takes a couple of hours.

Audrey hasn't called, so I will call her later.

The biggest emotional dilemma I have at the moment is how to take the next step with her. I am torn between my own grief, loss, and healing and doing what is right for her because you loved her. On the one hand, I want to read the eulogy at your funeral, and on the other, I just don't want to cause any animosity.

Audrey will never truly understand me or our relationship. However, I don't think it is right from a human perspective to blame her for that; it is certainly not right to punish her. I probably need to speak to her and just be honest. My concern: she rarely listens and already has an opinion; on top of that, she is now grieving, so it may be considered inappropriate on my behalf. However, there will always be criticism no matter what I do, so I may as well be true to myself. Forgive me if I get it wrong; it won't be out of malice.

6.52 p.m.

I have just spoken to Audrey. She is still very weepy, understandably.

It looks like your funeral will be next Thursday or Friday; she will confirm tomorrow. I have thanked her for what she has done for you and acknowledged that you were happy in your final years, recognising her for that.

I asked about reading your eulogy and was completely shut down. You did not want it, therefore I can't do it.

I can get past that, Dad. You led your life according to Audrey and Derek's rules, and the distance changed you, but I don't care. I loved you anyway. What is an eulogy? Only words, words that I can capture here and that are in my heart.

I will be travelling down and back up on the same day. I really don't want to socialise; it is not really a social event.

I need to finish now. Don't know how I feel and don't think it would be productive for me to write any more.

Goodnight, Dad.

3 September 2009
7.36 p.m.

Well, I am going to say this and maybe I will regret it; maybe I won't.

I have had a conversation with Audrey today about your funeral, date, and time communicated and documented.

In the high-pitched, breaking, and pathetic voice of the grieving widow, she has told me that she has booked one car (too expensive to have any more) and that she assumed Ange would be in her own car as she has the boys with her. I corrected her and told her that as my mum was coming, she could drive Ange's car and Ange WILL come with us in the main car.

The next knife wound: we can come and see your body at the funeral director's on the day of your funeral until 11.15 a.m. If we go to her house, she will come with us to see you. I have told her that Ange and I will come on our own to see our dad. Can she not even afford us this time together with you unchaperoned?

I know she is grieving and that she is upset, but please. I am trying so hard to ignore everything and give her the benefit of the doubt. I know she is trying to be nice, but everything feels like a dig, and she is not the only one grieving.

I really have never met anybody in my life that is so far away from self-awareness. It is such a gift to really know yourself, seek feedback, adapt your behaviour, and think of others before yourself, none of which Audrey seems to have the capacity to do. There is an inherent need to be the focal point – me, me, me! It feels like she is constantly seeking sympathy and telling a tale of woe in such a way that she cannot hear what others have to say. There seems to be little interest in opinions, inputs, or others' feelings.

Despite all of this, I try so hard to find gratitude and forgiveness. I am grateful for what she has done for you. I just don't want her to tell me what she has done for you every time we meet. It makes it all feel false, judgemental, and selfish.

I don't know how many times I have heard the story of how you could not get a pension because you had worked abroad and how she has had to support you financially. I thought it was for richer or for poorer?

Anyway, saying how I feel helps to remove the negative thoughts from my mind. I might settle now. Please, God, give me strength to forgive, forget, and be nice.

I have had a fairly normal day today, been to work, spoken to loads of people on the phone, been and sorted Ange out as she was having a bit of a crisis at the pub, came home, cooked the kids tea, and now talking to you.

No tears at all; it is strange. I feel so at peace for you, knowing you are in a better place. It is like any doubts I had before about life after death have gone completely. I have no fear, no doubts. It's like I know what is next all of a sudden. Weird. Do you think that is faith?

I know you were a bit sceptical, but you were such a good man that there really can be only one path for you to take, and I know you are on it.

I would love you to send me a sign that you are OK, maybe not today, but someday.

I think I might do some studying tonight. I haven't done any for over a week, and it will bring the sense of normality even closer.

One week to your funeral, and the closure of this chapter of my life. Surreal. I will not wonder or second-guess the future. I will just face it and myself as it arrives on a daily basis.

I was telling Shaun last night about the time you were fixing the wiring in an office and how you were up in the ceiling space when all of a sudden you fell through. All anyone could see were your two chubby legs dangling through the ceiling like Fred Flintstone's. That was before I was born, and the story has been told by everyone in the family. It must have been the funniest thing to see; Shaun and I had a giggle. You were the clumsiest man I have ever known. I always knew you had been by the coffee stains on my carpet and various items of broken furniture. I would do anything now to see coffee stains on my cream carpet, because what do stains matter in the big scale of things?

Your clumsiness was endearing; you were endearing. I bet you are making a right mess in heaven right now, and God is rolling his eyes just like Mum used to do.

I have one life and one chance to make it count for something... I'm free to choose what that something is, and the something I've chosen is my faith. Now, my faith goes beyond theology and religion and requires considerable work and effort. My faith demands – this is not optional – my faith demands that I do whatever I can, wherever I am, whenever I can, for as long as I can with whatever I have to try to make a difference.
Jimmy Carter

4 September 2009
11.19 p.m.

Just in from work and sat and had some supper with Shaun. He is just taking the dogs for a walk while I talk to you.

I am getting organised again.

I realised today how disorganised I have been over the last month when an unpaid bill appeared. I never miss a payment on anything.

I went through my in-tray and realised I have been putting things off for weeks. So next week I am going to focus on short-term goals and organisation and planning.

I have been thinking about you constantly, but during

that drive home from work, it is like I have your name and face on repeat all the way home. The thoughts are so intense, desperately seeking a sign that you are OK. Very close to tears on the way home tonight, but I did not give in.

I have booked a facial for Tuesday in the vain attempt to try and make myself look half decent for your funeral. Why? Can't answer that. Maybe I will feel better, and it will help me get through the day. I certainly couldn't look any worse. My eyes look so sad and wrinkled. It is hard to feel good when I have lost you, and I really want the sadness to lift.

I am getting on with my life. Nobody would guess I am so sad as I am in control and being strong for everyone. But I am so, so sad because I can't see you. I know I will see you again, but I want to see you now.

I feel like Verruca Salt's in Willy Wonka and the Chocolate Factory "I Want It Now"!!

I am not writing any more tonight. I am tired and want to wind down a bit, so I am going to watch a bit of TV.

I love you and miss you, Mr Brian King. I will speak to you again tomorrow.

Goodnight.

Where you used to be,
There is a hole in the world,

Which I find myself constantly
Walking around in the daytime,
And falling in at night.
I miss you like hell.
Edna St. Vincent Millay

5 September 2009
9.32 a.m.

I just received an e-mail from Hilary. She is so lovely and caring, and I just don't understand why you cut her out of your life. It was the same with Ange. She is such a lovely person, ditsy and rubbish with money, but lovely. Your sister and your daughter, why? Is it because you didn't want to get hurt? You were so critical of both of them. But I still don't think that was you. I think it was the repetition of unforgiving comments you heard constantly from your companions.

You will have to tell me when we meet again.

I am never going to do that with any member of my family. Maybe it was to teach me that lesson that you did it. Harsh.

As you can probably guess, I woke up thinking about you. Hence the early comments. Then Hilary's e-mail made me cry, so I thought I had better have a word with you.

I hope that when you are reviewing your life, you learn from your errors in judgement and can take on responsibility and forgive yourself. I think Ange has definitely learned her lesson and will not be stubborn again as long as she lives. That is part of your legacy, so thanks for that.

I am going downstairs for a cuppa and some breakfast now, and I am just going to enjoy my wonderful family and tell them all how much I love them.

I feel you are with me, Dad, enjoy spending time with me like I always did with you.

Speak later.

10.36 p.m.

Love is the answer to everything.

The only way you can prevail, survive, and thrive is to love.

Hate, anger, and depression just fester away at your soul and make it

visible that you are not a good person.

We all have the capacity to hate, and to live in anger, but we also have the ability to choose to love, to be kind, to be worthy of this life.

I choose love.

I will not be angry at Audrey no matter how hurtful her words. I will rise above it and be kind to her anyway.

This I will do for you and also for me.

You have taken me on a journey these last six weeks, Dad, an emotional roller coaster of a journey, but I was ready and a willing participant.

Thank you so much for the lesson. I can take this forward with me for the rest of my life.

I feel good about the future having been equipped with so much knowledge this year. Learning is out there every day for us all, the only thing we have to do is open our eyes, ears, minds, and hearts.

My life is full of wonderful people, and I am so grateful for each and every one. You are one of them, as I consider you to be with me all the time. What a wonderful life.

Am I full of it tonight or what?

Anyway, that is how I am feeling tonight and from this day forth. Honesty is what I committed to and that is what you will get. If you were still here, you would run a mile if I said all of that to you; now you have to listen to me.

With those thoughts in my head, I am going to sleep and dream of you.

Goodnight, Dad. Sleep tight.

An individual has not started living until he can rise above the narrow confines of his individualistic concerns to the broader concerns of all humanity.
Martin Luther King, Jr

6 September 2009
7.36 p.m.

I have spent the day with a very special lady today in the hope of creating the solution for Ange in the pub. Ange is struggling on her own trying to juggle everything, so I approached the lovely Tracie to see if she would be interested in the partnership. I think it may be a goer and the right solution for all.

I am looking after her, Dad, like I always have; you don't have to be concerned.

I need to see what I can do for Nathan as well; he needs some support at the minute.

Sometimes it is hard being all things to all people, especially when I have so much to do for myself. But life is a challenge, and it is our duty to rise to it, no matter what.

I am looking forward to getting stuck in writing and studying again next week when the kids are back to school.

It is four days to your funeral, and I can't say I am looking forward to that one little bit. I intend to be strong, be there for others, and survive the day, which is the best I can offer.

I have written a card for Audrey offering her love, gratitude, and forgiveness and wrapped a gift for her that I think will help. I promised to be kind and live in love, not hate, so that is what I am doing.

I am so tired tonight. I am hoping that I can settle back into a more normal sleep pattern after Thursday.

I also need to chase my new date for my operation. I can't afford for that to drag on; the sooner the better.

Goodness me, we have just had Sheena and Viv on the phone, one crying the other one shouting. Do they not realise that we are grieving at the minute? What a time to bring their arguments into our lives and what a waste of energy arguing over who said what and when. What does it all matter? I would give my last penny to have you back in my life for just an hour, and they are arguing over something that was said! Life is too damn short, and it has upset me. *No more arguments!* Shaun was a bit firm with Sheena on the phone. He has had enough of the pettiness too. He doesn't even know what Viv was screaming about, and she told him to f*** off when he said he wasn't interested.

Why do people do that?

What is the point of hurting one another?

How selfish!

I can't ever remember us ever disagreeing, let alone using harsh words.

You were so lovely, and I love you for that.

I choose love.

God grant me the serenity to accept the people I cannot change, the courage to change the one I can, and the wisdom to know it's me.
Author unknown

7 September 2009
1.57 p.m.

Oh, Dad, I sent Audrey a text this morning to see how she was and let her know I was thinking about her. Her response said, "totally heartbroken." I know how she feels. The only difference is, I still have my family, but she will be alone. Not a great place to be when you have lost somebody you love.

I know she has lots of friends, but I am sure that there will be a void where you used to be, and there lies the part of me that finds it impossible to be anything but non-judgemental, empathetic, and understanding. I will not be able to help myself in offering the olive branch, no matter how much hurt I have encountered from her words. Maybe she will learn something from having you, interacting with me, and reading this diary.

I think that there is potential for her to behave in a better way, but some learning about her impact on others is essential.

At this point, though, despite all of my anger and disappointment in her sheer lack of understanding of my pain and her impact on it, I can definitely forgive and forget.

If I can put up with Sheena and Viv behaving badly and still find forgiveness and love, then I can do it for Audrey.

Anyway, I took Becca, Dan, and Emma to the Lion's Den and to Sprinkles for a big milkshake today. Becca is back at school tomorrow, and I wanted a bit of time with them that was happy.

Just thought I would have a brief chat before work. It will be straight to bed when I get in because I will be up at 6.00 a.m. to be back in school run routine.

Becca has been seeing signs that you are with us everywhere, and she has been talking to you and praying for you. I hope you heard. Having that sort of unshakable belief is a big comfort to her and should be a lesson to all adults.

I feel a bit angry today. I don't know what I am angry about. Nothing in particular? It is hard not to take it out on the kids when they are shouting at each other. That problem will resolve itself tomorrow when Becca is back at school.

Who would have believed that the week before the school holidays started was when you were diagnosed with cancer? And now you are gone. Sometimes I am just at a loss for words.

Only three days until our final goodbye. I feel cold and tired.

We must care about the world of our children and

grandchildren, a world we may never see.
Bertrand Russell

10.42 p.m.

I know I said I was going straight to bed, but I am having a bad day and need to talk to you. I found myself sobbing just because you were gone, for the first time in a week. I think that maybe the sheer futility of the behaviour between Sheena and Viv last night hit me today. Why would you treat a parent like that? Why would you scream and shout at your brother for no reason? Depression is not an excuse. We all have the ability to choose our behaviour even if we feel low.

I will never understand why loved ones treat each other this way. I have never felt the need to behave like that; it's like they just do not have the ability to learn. Have we lost the ability to just love and support each other? There seems to be a daily occurrence now of hate and violence, be it words or physical. Why is everyone so angry?

We are ruining our planet, killing animals and each other, finding new atrocities every day, and meddling with our food so it no longer has any nutritional value. We have just lost faith!

Boy, where did that come from? Maybe I need to become an activist and fight for something. Just kidding. I need to do what I planned and help others really get to know themselves and be all they can be; that will be my legacy.

I feel better after talking to you, and the tears have gone. Thanks, Dad.

I quote others only in order the better to express myself.
Michel de Montaigne

8 September 2009
8.17 p.m.

I have had such an odd day. I really think that the behaviour that Sheena and Viv demonstrated the other night has knocked me for six. I have been weepy and just don't feel right. I sent Shaun out for a bottle of Asti and a Chinese tonight. So now I am comfort eating. Well, if I am totally honest, I have been doing that for a week!

I had to phone Ange and apologise tonight. I was a bit full on with her today, having a go at Gary and just being me! Anyway, at least I had the balls to pick up the phone and say sorry and I love you. She knows what I am like better than anyone except Shaun actually.

Shaun and I have just sat and chatted over Asti and Chinese and had a few tears. I am so lucky to have him. He is my soulmate, and I love every minute with him, even when we are bickering.

I have not been very nice to the kids today. I think I just need a bit of me time, but it is very hard to get. It's not their fault, and I need to make up for it tomorrow.

Well, I had my facial this morning, and then I have had a weepy day, so the benefits have probably been washed away. You will just have to take me as I am, but then you always did, didn't you?

I am finding it harder to write, the closer it gets to your funeral. It's almost like dread that after Thursday, there will be nothing. At the moment, your funeral is pending. Then what? I don't want to say goodbye. It sounds daft when that is what I did the week before you died, but that is how I feel today. I won't have you. The diary will be finished and... I can't even describe it. It is more than emptiness; it goes deeper.

I have been experiencing flashbacks for the last two days. Somebody will say something, and an image of you and me pops into my head. For instance, somebody said something about Wooler yesterday, and Yearle House, and you came back to me. It was a particular moment in the kitchen with Dougal, the daft dog, and it felt so real and so intense. Then it was gone, and I felt loss.

It's funny, though, that in every image, you are laughing – a good hearty laugh with a smile so broad it covers your entire face.

I loved your laugh. You didn't seem to do it as often over the past few years; you always seemed more serious. Not when the kids were there, though. Becca made you laugh like I used too. Oh my goodness, lots of flashbacks of how you looked at Becca. You really loved her, like you loved me. I don't know if I noticed every look at the time, but they seem to be stored in my memory. Thank you, thank you, thank you.

Now I am sobbing again and typing through the tears. Sixty-seven is just too young. I wanted you longer. It sounds so selfish, but I can't help it.

I know there are many young people who die, and I cannot imagine the pain of that. It must be the most terrible pain on earth to endure. However, all loss is painful, and when it happens to you, it is your pain. Nobody else can feel it nor understand it as it is personal. We can all empathise and feel emotion when others lose loved ones, but the reality of your own loss is about you and your memories. Ralph Waldo Emerson articulates it well when he comments on the loss of his son: "My son, a perfect little boy of five years and three months, had ended his earthly life. You can never sympathize with me; you can never know how much of me such a young child can take away. A few weeks ago I accounted myself a very rich man, and now the poorest of all."

The loss of someone you love so much can erase all meaning from any possession or desire. It can give you a sense of the meaningless, yet it can also give you a sense of purpose, for we will all die, and until we do, we need to be useful.

I will be fine tomorrow, Dad. You can't be strong

24/7. I am entitled to my bad days. I just lost someone who meant the world to me, and now my world has changed.

I just need a hug tonight.

Pain and death are part of life. To reject them is to reject life itself.
Havelock Ellis

9 September 2009
10.00 a.m.

I feel much better today.

I was up at 6.00 a.m., and Becca and I took the dogs for a long walk. I had breakfast with her and made up for yesterday.

Dan is back to school today as well, so I have that time to myself I wanted yesterday, and guess what, not so keen on it now I have it!

I am going to Amanda's for coffee in about half an hour, then in to Alnwick to see the bank manager about the pub. I have done most of the ironing, tidied up, put the washing on and am just having a coffee and talking to you.

It is your funeral tomorrow, and I really need to get myself to a good place today. I want to be strong and supportive, not weepy and needy.

I have laid all of our clothes out ready because we are leaving at 6.45 a.m. I have some photographs of you to pick up today while I am in Alnwick. I had copies made for Ange, Nathan, and Jack.

Now all I need to achieve is an early night and a good night's sleep. Help me out with that, Dad, as I am still not sleeping well.

I will probably not write tonight as I need to focus. I may meditate for an hour to properly relax and help with sleep.

It will be a long day tomorrow, so my next entry will be Friday, 11 September – goodness me, 9/11. I will write my final comments on a day that so many innocent people lost their lives needlessly.

I will remember them and you and say a prayer for all of you.

I am signing off now, Dad. I will talk to you still, don't worry. Your funeral may be the end of this diary, but it will never stop me talking to you.

How much I love you is difficult for me to express in words; how much I miss you even harder. But the smile on my face when I think about you and remember is visible for all to see.

If you smile when no one else is around, you really mean it.
Andy Rooney

Or, in the very famous and inspirational words of Charlie Chaplin:

Smile though your heart is aching
Smile even though it's breaking
When there are clouds in the sky, you'll get by
If you smile through your fear and sorrow
Smile and maybe tomorrow
You'll see the sun come shining through for you
Light up your face with gladness
Hide every trace of sadness
Although a tear may be ever so near
That's the time you must keep on trying
Smile, what's the use of crying?
You'll find that life is still worthwhile
If you just smile

9/11 – **11 September 2009**
12.55 p.m.

For all of those who died, my thoughts are with you and with your families; this day must serve as a painful annual reminder of the enormity of their loss.

For you, Dad, I will remember you every year on 1st September, the day you left me, and again on this day, the day I completed my diary.

Yesterday was hard.

I did not cry, but it was hard.

We set off at 6.45 a.m. and arrived to meet Ange, Elaine, and the boys at 10.30 a.m. Mum and I talked about you fondly in the car. Memories, so many happy memories. Ange and I went to Audrey's to check in and get the directions to the funeral director's. And yes, we had to suffer many more hurtful comments in the short time we were there, but I have decided that it serves no purpose to publish them. Needless to say, they continued throughout the day.

Audrey was obviously distraught. We gave her a hug and then came to see you.

There are no words to describe the feeling of going to see the body of your parent. It was not you, it was just a body – your spirit long gone to a much better place. I was able to draw strength from my beliefs and faith at that moment. I am not getting all religious on you, Dad. I just know for sure you are somewhere better.

Ange was very upset, and I found it hard to comfort her. After all, her grief is as personal to her as mine is to me.

We left you and went back to the hotel to wait for Caroline and Nick.

Cheryl was there when we arrived, and we all sat outside in the sunshine chatting about you and enjoying the time. You would have loved to have been there with us with a pint in one hand and a cigar in the other.

Caroline and Nick arrived at about twelve and joined us. It must have been a bit full on for Caroline. Seven weeks ago she had only a few family; now she has inherited the munsters! You can pick your friends, but why would you want to when you can spend time with a motley crew like us?

We headed to your house at 12.30 p.m. to join the cortege. Ange and I were going in the funeral car with Audrey, Derek, their mum, and Audrey's friend Beryl. Draw your own conclusions from that.

Prior to the car's arriving, Audrey was emotionally distraught and very dramatic with it, virtually throwing herself to the ground and screaming out loud as the hearse arrived with you in it. She who cries the loudest loves you the most?

We followed you to the crematorium, and, without any let up, the sobbing continued. Not your girls, though. We were strong for you, Dad.

The service was basic to say the least. We had no input, so there was no mention of any memories or times before Audrey. Complete control. Although you had stated that you did not want any fuss or music, there were flowers from Audrey and Freddie (the dog), there was music, and there was fuss. You also stated you did not want an eulogy, so I did not have that once-in-a-lifetime opportunity to pay tribute to my wonderful, special dad.

Flowers from Audrey – yes. Flowers from the dog – yes. Music selected by Audrey – yes. Information about you from Audrey – yes. Eulogy from your loving daughter – no chance! You were also acknowledged as being a loving husband, father, grandad, friend, and colleague. No mention of being a brother or uncle – and there goes another knife wound.

Stripped of all of this, I managed not to shed a tear during the charade that was attended by so many people I did not know.

After the service, I gathered your family – Ange, Nathan, Jack, Shaun, Becca, Mum, Cheryl, Elaine, Caroline, Nick, and me representing Hilary in Australia – and read your eulogy in the car park. This was the only point of the day that I came anywhere near to tears, as these were heartfelt words written by your biggest fan!

We then met up with the other guests at the hotel and stayed for an appropriate time before leaving.

And that is it, Dad.

To steal a phrase from Homer J Simpson, it was "the worst day of my life so far".

Today I was up at 6.00 a.m. and took the dogs out for an hour on the same route as we had walked in April of this year. I cried almost the whole time, for no other reason than I miss you. I love you, and I am exhausted from compromising.

I do not want any more pain, hurtful comments, snide remarks, opinions, digs, or misguided and uneducated wisdom!

I have had enough.

I just want my happy memories of you – they were all happy – and to get on with my life.

I know you will be with me and that you will forgive

me when I can't find the strength to deal with Audrey and give me strength when I have to. I just need a bit of time to grieve.

I can deal with anyone and anything else, but for the moment, not her.

I will find the strength again, I promise you.

Cancer has taken you from me to somewhere better.

Your earthly journey has ended, and a new and exciting time for you begins. Enjoy your new home. Remember how much you were loved on earth, and prepare my path for when the time comes.

Oh my goodness, floods of tears.

My dad.

My daft, lovely dad.

I love you.

In This Farewell

In this farewell...
There is no weakness
For you taught me well
There is confidence and strength
For I will try not to cry, but I won't apologise if I do

In this farewell...
There is no disappointment
For how many of us are perfect?
There is acceptance
For in accepting responsibility for everything in our
life, we give ourselves the opportunity to grow

In this farewell...
There are no tears of regret
For all that needed to be said was said
There are tears of sadness
For the loss of a wonderful and loving man, who I
was proud to call Dad

In this farewell...
There is no bitterness or anger
For all of us there will be an end
There is gratitude and joy
For the world was a better place with you in it, you
brought laughter, a great gift in the memory of
those who loved you

In this farewell...
There is no loss
For you have suffered enough
There is hope
For your early departure may inspire others to raise
money for cancer research so that they may see a
cure. You can rely on me, Dad

In this farewell...
There is no blame or resentment
For what would be the point?
There is togetherness and family unity
For you did a wonderful thing in your final months
without even knowing, you brought together those
loved but lost. A credible legacy

In this farewell...
There is no fear
For I have never seen a braver man
There is courage and motivation
For you inspired me in life to be who I am, and you
inspired me in death to face the world no matter
what

In this farewell...
There is no despair
For you found happiness in your final years
There is recognition
For I am grateful for your happiness

In this farewell...
There is a little girl

Staring at a coffin
Longing for one last hug
Knowing it is too late

So, in this farewell…
There is one last request
Meet me when my time comes
And know I will think about you every day till then.

Farewell, Dad. God speed.

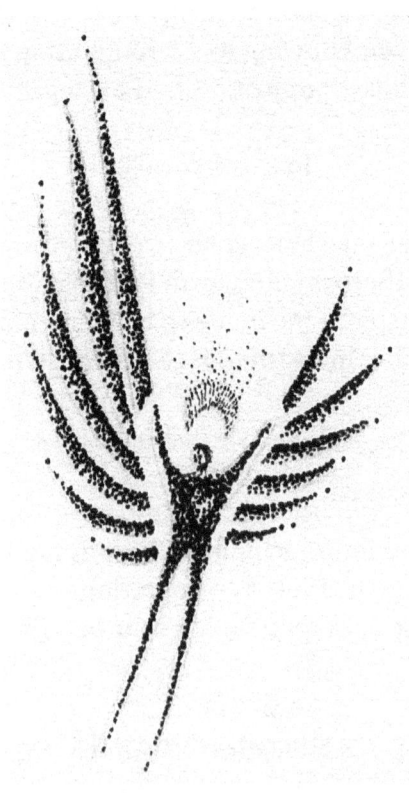

About the Author

A. J. King like many others in the UK had spent her life working hard, progressing through the ranks to a senior management level. But 2009 had different plans for her that would explode over a six month period changing life as she knew it.

At 44 years old, with two young children, a happy marriage and a great job, things seemed to be bordering on perfect, then one Sunday morning in March a freak event caused a serious car crash on her way to work resulting in a month off. Having reflection time and she made a big decision to leave her career behind and do something new.

Being a 'glass half full' type of person she booked herself on some courses and set about planning her own business with enthusiasm. She called a friend and took a part time job to keep the wolves from the door.

In June she collapsed at work and was rushed to hospital for the second time, another month off work followed and so did major surgery. During this period she completed two diplomas and signed up for a degree. And just as she was getting ready to return to work she made a phone call that would start a whirlwind of change and emotion.

Her dad was diagnosed with terminal cancer, she knew instantly that if she did not do something positive with this experience then it may all be just too much, so the night of the call was the night she started a diary that would teach her more about life and love than you could learn in a lifetime.